400 MCQS IN PAEDIATRICS FOR MRCPCH PART I

D0235115

To my father Giumma, my mother Salema, brothers Omran, Abdulazeez, Ibrahim, and sisters Saaida, Kadiga, Zuhra, Taliga and Hamida who encouraged and supported me until I finished medical school and higher education in Libya and the UK.

400 MCQS IN PAEDIATRICS FOR MRCPCH PART I

By

Nagi Giumma Barakat
MB BCh MRCPCH MSc epilepsy CCST
St Thomas' Hospital
Lambeth Palace Road
London

Reviewed by
Colin M Stern
Consultant Paediatrician
St Thomas' Hospital
Lambeth Palace Road
London

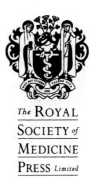

The ROYAL
SOCIETY of
MEDICINE
PRESS Limited

© 2001 Royal Society of Medicine Press Ltd
1 Wimpole Street, London W1G 0AE
207 Westminster Road, Lake Forest IL 60045 USA
www.rsmpress.co.uk

British Library Cataloguing in Publication Data
A catalogue record for this book is available from the British Library

ISBN: 1–85315–491–1

Typeset by Phoenix Photosetting, Chatham, Kent

Printed in Great Britain by Bell and Bain Ltd, Glasgow

Contents

Foreword

Dr Nagi Barakat has produced, in his third collection of Multiple Choice Questions, another valuable resource for the paediatric postgraduate student who is seeking to hone his knowledge in preparation for Part I of the MRCPCH examination. Dr Barakat is an experienced postgraduate tutor who has considerable understanding of the pitfalls that await the unwary examination candidate and his questions explore many of the thornier questions that may be asked.

It takes much time and patience to collate such a broad range of subjects and to anotate the answers so that ambiguity, while an essential constituent and a probing question on the one hand, is restrained within the context of the reasonable doubt, on the other. A student alone can study a book such as this but, when its contents are discussed with a colleague, it has the benefit of both broadening debate and crystallising understanding, while at the same time, challenging current understanding.

I am certain that this collection is a valuable addition to the armamentarium of the prospective paediatrician.

Colin Stern

Preface

The paediatric option of the MRCPCH [UK] Part 1 examination was introduced in October 1993, necessitating an MCQ book focusing more specifically on paediatric topics. Each chapter in this book contains questions designed to test candidates' knowledge of the basic sciences as well as clinical conditions. Areas covered include molecular biology, biochemistry, physiology, microbiology, pathology, immunology, pharmacology and statistics.

This is my third book for candidates who are preparing for MRCPCH parts I and II. My first book, *MCQs in Paediatrics for MRCP Part I*, was published in June 1994 and has sold more than 4000 copies. This book is completely different and is more clinically oriented. This book and my other book are complementary to each other.

I wish to thank all my colleagues, former teachers and examiners who have unwittingly provided ideas for many of the questions. In addition, Dr Colin M Stern has provided a great deal of support and help in the preparation of this text. My wife, Lobna Maktari supported me and was very helpful.

NGB
London
June 2001

Acknowledgement

I am very grateful to my wife and family, Dr C M Stern, and Mr Peter Richardson from The Royal Society of Medicine who supported me and helped me to finish this book. Many thanks to Nora Naughton, Sam Gear and Ruth Swan who edited this and my previous book. Thank you to all of you.

NGB
London 2001

The MRCPCH Part I examination

The examination is a multiple choice question paper consisting of 60 questions. The multiple choice questions are designed to test the candidate's reasoning ability as well as knowledge of basic facts. Each question consists of a stem statement with five following items. The candidate has to answer all questions with "true" or "false". It is important to read the stem and items carefully, but answer each item independently, disregarding the other statements in the question. The answer sheets are read by an automatic document reader so mark the answer paper boldly and clearly. If you change your answer, erase it carefully and re-mark the paper.

On your first run through of the examination paper, either mark the answers in the question paper or straight onto the paper. Leave enough time at the end to go over your answers and check that the answer sheet is correctly marked. Try again to answer any difficult questions but avoid repeated reviews as this is usually counter-productive.

The examination is no longer negatively marked. The pass mark will vary, but in general you should aim to answer all the questions.

Preparing for the examination

It is important to achieve a good knowledge of the basic sciences relevant to clinical paediatrics. The recommended texts are useful, but also try to attend a course specifically designed for the paediatric Part 1 examination. Once you have acquired the basic knowledge, start to do as many MCQs as you can, aiming to score over 80% correct.

MCQ examination technique

It is important to accept the questions at face value and not to look for hidden meanings or ambiguities. Try to avoid genuine guessing but at the same time do not give in too easily and try to reason through the question without spending too long on the problem. If you are fairly certain of the answer, commit yourself on the answer sheet and record "true" or "false".

The wording of MCQs may present some difficulty and the meaning of many terms is outlined in the following table. Be wary of universal statements such as "only", "never", "invariably", and "always", which are usually false.

Terminology used in MCQs

Always	There are no recognised exceptions
Never	
Can be	Reported [or recognised] to occur
May be	
Occurs	No statement of frequency
Commonly	An occurrence rate of greater than 50%
Frequently	
Likely	
Often	
Characteristic	Features that occur frequently enough to be of
Typical	diagnostic significance although they are not pathognomonic
Specific	A feature that occurs only in the named disease
Pathognomonic	and no other
Recognised feature	It has been reported to be a feature or association

In summary, the best preparation for the examination is a combination of knowledge and plenty of MCQ practice including past papers. If you are well prepared you are likely to pass, but remember that most members of the Royal College of Paediatrics and Child Health will have failed some part of the exam on at least one occasion.

Recommended texts and references

Aicardi J. (1998) *Childhood Nervous System Diseases*, 2nd edn. Mac Keith Press, London.

Behrman R.E., Kleigman R.M., Nelson W.E., and Vaughan V.C. (2000) *Nelson's Textbook of Paediatrics*, 16th edn. W.B. Saunders, London.

BMJ (1999) *Advanced Paediatric Life Support, the Practical Approach*, 3rd edn. BMJ Publishing Group, London.

Campbell A.G.M. & McIntosh N. (1998) *Forfar's Textbook of Paediatrics*, 5th edn. Churchill Livingstone, Edinburgh.

David T.J. (1999, 2000) *Recent Advances in Paediatrics* 15 and 16. Churchill Livingstone, Edinburgh.

Fenichel G.M. (1993) *Clinical Pediatric Neurology—a Signs and Symptoms Approach*, 2nd edn. W.B. Saunders, London.

Illingworth R.S. (1987) *The Development of Infants and Young Children*, 8th edn. Churchill Livingstone, Edinburgh.

Department of Health, UK (1992 edn) *Immunisation against Infectious Disease*, HMSO.

Postlethwaite R.J. (1986) *Clinical Paediatric Nephrology*, 1st edn. IOP Publishing Limited, Bristol.

Archives of Disease in Childhood (1995–2000). Royal College of Paediatrics and Child Health, London.

Roberton M. (1992) Textbook of Neonatology, 2nd edn. Churchill Livingstone, Edinburgh.

Neonatology questions

Question 1

Indications for foetal blood sampling include

A Early deceleration
B Passage of meconium
C Abnormal foetal heart sound
D Following acceleration of labour by oxytocin
E Severe deceleration

Question 2

Systems which develop from the ectoderm include

A Brain and neural tube
B Limbs
C Cardiovascular system
D Gastrointestinal system
E Face

Question 3

Are the following statements about embryonic growth true or false?

A The embryonic period refers to the period from conception to delivery
B The embryo can be detected by US 28 days after conception
C During the embryonic period the conceptus is 30 mm in length
D During the foetal period the foetus grows at about 1.5 cm/week
E The heart starts to beat at 12 weeks from LMP

Question 4

Are the following statements about birth trauma true or false?

A Subconjunctival haemorrhage is common
B Caput succedaneum is subcutaneous effusion due to laceration of blood vessels
C Cephalhaematoma is limited by the cranial bones
D VIIth nerve cranial palsy always requires surgical decompression
E Klumpke's palsy results from a lesion at C5–6

Question 5

Newborn babies with moderate hypoxic ischaemic encephalopathy (HIE) may have

A Seizures
B Weak suck
C Lethargy
D Tone greater in arms than in legs
E Need for respiratory support

Question 6

Seizures following hypoxic ischaemic encephalopathy can be treated with

A ACTH
B Phenobarbitone
C Lignocaine
D Thiopentone
E Diazepam

Question 7

Are the following statements about RDS true or false?

A Ground glass appearance on CXR is pathognomonic
B Mixed respiratory and metabolic acidosis is a common finding
C Increase in oxygen requirement after 2–3 days is an indication of worsening of RDS
D Glucocorticoids reduce the severity of RDS if given early to premature babies with risk factors
E Three doses of surfactant are always needed

Question 8

Are the following statements about CPAP used in RDS true or false?

A Prevents alveolar collapse during expiration
B Can be used in smaller babies
C Used in acute collapse
D Used to keep Pao_2 between 8 and 10 KPa
E Can be used in weaning from IPPV

Question 9

Recognised complications of surfactant therapy in RDS include

A Pulmonary haemorrhage
B Bronchopulmonary dysplasia
C Increased incidence of patent ductus arteriosus
D Intraventricular haemorrhage
E Infection

Question 10

Are the following statements about apnoeic attack in neonates true or false?

A More common in babies with a respiratory problem than in those with a neurological problem
B Characterised by cessation of respiration for >40 s
C Can be caused by necrotising enterocolitis
D Central apnoea is characterised by cessation of respiratory effort and airflow
E There is a strong association between obstructive apnoea and SIDS

Question 11

Problems associated more with a term baby than one that is small for gestational age include

A Hypoglycaemia
B Infection
C Hypoxia
D Polycythaemia
E Intraventricular haemorrhage

Question 12

Contraindications to the use of indomethacin in preterm and term infants with PDA are

A Creatinine >60 mmol/l
B Bleeding disorders
C Intracranial haemorrhage within the preceding 3 weeks
D Necrotising enterocolitis
E Total urine output of <2 ml/kg/h

Question 13

Are the following statements about ECG findings in congenital heart defect true or false?

A TAPV with pulmonary valve obstruction—RAH
B Tricuspid atresia—superior axis deviation
C TOF—RVH
D Ebstein's anomaly—LBBB
E D-TGA with intact ventricular septum—RVH is severe

Question 14

Conjugated hyperbilirubinaemia at the age of 2 weeks may be due to

A Hypothyroidism
B Dubin–Johnson syndrome
C Pyloric stenosis
D Choledochal cyst
E Gilbert's syndrome

Question 15

Low platelet count in a healthy 5-day-old infant is commonly due to

A Maternal idiopathic thrombocytopenic purpura
B Kasabach–Merritt syndrome
C Hydralazine
D Bernard–Soulier syndrome
E Isoimmune thrombocytopenia

Question 16

Are the following statements true or false?

A PVL is a small cyst secondary to IVH
B Antepartum haemorrhage is a known risk factor in PVL
C Cerebellar haemorrhage has a good outcome
D Thalamic haemorrhage arises from the choroidal plexus
E Few infants develop cerebral palsy after PVL

Question 17

Common aetiologies of acute renal failure in newborn infants include

A Polycythaemia
B Renal vein thrombosis following asphyxia
C Urinary obstruction
D Haemorrhage
E Sepsis

Question 18

Common late manifestations of congenital rubella infection include

A Interstitial pneumonitis
B Diabetes mellitus
C Cataract
D Autism
E Retinopathy

Question 19

Common causes of haematuria in newborn babies include

A Urinary tract infection
B Renal vein thrombosis
C Congenital nephrotic syndrome
D Coagulation defects
E Nephritis secondary to congenital CMV infection

Question 20

Risk factors predisposing to retinopathy of prematurity include

A Blood transfusion
B Consistently high P_{O_2}
C High pH
D Low vitamin E
E Low P_{CO_2}

Question 21

Are the following statements about immunity in newborn babies true or false?

A IgG starts to cross the placenta as early as 32 weeks of gestation
B IgM starts to cross at 36–37 weeks of gestation
C IgG_2 is higher than IgG_4
D 50% of complement is present
E T-cell counts are depressed by hyperbilirubinaemia

Question 22

Diagnostic tests for congenital infections in newborn babies include

A Urine—CMV
B Immune fluorescence—chicken pox
C Immune fluorescence IgM test—toxoplasmosis
D HIV—positive HIV antibody
E HBsAg + HBc antibody—hepatitis B infection

Question 23

Are the following statements about hypoglycaemia in the neonatal period true or false?

A The blood glucose level adopted for diagnosing hypoglycaemia is 2.5 mmol/l
B In IUGR both glycogenolysis and gluconeogenesis are limited in activity
C The brain cannot use ketones and lactate as substitutes for glucose
D 5 ml of 10% dextrose is used as treatment of profound hypoglycaemia
E Insulin receptors are decreased in the infant of a diabetic mother

Question 24

Drugs that induce hypoglycaemia in the newborn infant if taken by the mother include

A Atenolol
B Diazoxide
C Thiazides
D Amoxycillin
E Dexamethasone

Question 25

Laboratory findings in rickets of prematurity in a breast-fed baby include

A High alkaline phosphatase
B Normal phosphorus level
C Hyperphosphaturia
D Hypocalcaemia
E Hypercalciuria

Genetics questions

Question 26

Are the following statements about chromosomes true or false?

A Each nucleolus contains 46 chromosomes
B Deoxyribonucleoprotein is the basic unit of the chromosome
C A mutation results when a segment of DNA on one chromosome joins with another segment that is normally located
D A mutation does not disturb cell function
E On fertilisation the spermatocyte carries mitochondria into the oocyte

Question 27

Are the following linkages between childhood disorders and chromosomal locations true or false?

A Cystic fibrosis—7
B Duchenne muscular dystrophy—Xp21
C Fragile X syndrome—Xq27
D Thalassaemia—17
E Retinoblastoma—13

Question 28

Which of the following are X-linked recessive inherited diseases?

A Asphyxiating thoracic dystrophy of Jeune
B Cartilage–hair hypoplasia
C Anhidrotic ectodermal dysplasia
D Christmas disease
E Ocular albinism

Question 29

Characteristic features of autosomal recessive inherited diseases include

A 50% risk of recurrence
B Both parents normal
C More males affected
D All children of homozygous parents are heterozygous
E Affected individual born in one family generation only

Question 30

Common features of systemic involvement in Down's syndrome include

A Eyes—myopia
B Skeletal—frequent fractures
C GI tract—constipation
D Gonads—low fertility in males
E CNS—1–5% have epilepsy

Question 31

Features more commonly associated with trisomy 13 than trisomy 18 are

A Rocker bottom feet
B Colobomata
C Patent ductus arteriosus
D Horse shoe kidney
E Cleft lip and palate

Question 32

Common teratogenic drugs include

A Aminopterin
B Phenytoin
C Aspirin
D Heparin
E Tetracycline

Question 33

Are the following linkages between causes and abnormalities true or false?

A Alcoholism—growth retardation
B Cigarette smoking—mental retardation
C Diabetes mellitus—skeletal deformity
D Phenylketonuria—microcephaly
E Marijuana smoking—bleeding problem

Question 34

Are the following linkages between intra-uterine infection and abnormality in the newborn baby true or false?

A Cytomegalovirus—macrocephaly
B Rubella—cataract
C Herpes simplex—skeletal deformity
D Parvovirus—anaemia
E Toxoplasmosis—deafness

Question 35

The following are commonly associated with mental retardation

A Angleman syndrome
B Marden–Walker syndrome
C Crouzon syndrome
D Morquio syndrome
E Silver–Russell syndrome

Question 36

Macroglossia is a common feature of

A Hurler syndrome
B Seckel "bird-headed dwarf" syndrome
C Beckwith–Wiedemann syndrome
D Cretinism
E Down's syndrome

Question 37

Obesity is a common feature of

A Laurence–Moon–Biedl syndrome
B Goldenhaar syndrome
C Progeria
D Cohen syndrome
E Prader–Willi syndrome

Question 38

Syndromes commonly associated with cleft palate

A Stickler–Marshall
B Edwards' (trisomy 18)
C Van der Woude
D Holoprosencephaly
E Can be familial

Question 39

Are the following statements about neural tube defects in children true or false?

A Risk of recurrence after one affected child is 4%
B Risk of recurrence after two affected children is 20%
C More than 90% can be diagnosed antenatally by alpha-fetoprotein and ultrasound
D Meningomyelocele is not compatible with life
E Diastematomyelia is a consequence of neural tube defect

Question 40

Retinitis pigmentosa is a common feature of

A Refsum syndrome
B Sturge–Weber syndrome
C Toxoplasmosis
D Tuberous sclerosis
E Abetalipoproteinaemia

Question 41

The following anomalies are associated with Noonan's syndrome

A Coarctation of aorta
B Widely spaced nipples
C Males are sterile
D Lymphoedema
E Inherited as autosomal recessive

Growth, development and puberty questions

Question 42

The prenatal and perinatal factors that affect developmental assessment are

A Parental education
B Illegitimacy
C Multiple pregnancy
D Nutritional status
E Drugs used by mother

Question 43

Factors that may affect the development of children include

A Adoption
B Small family
C Fostering
D Emotional deprivation
E Lack of stimulation

Question 44

A 3-month-old infant can

A Keep its head in the midline/erect on sitting
B Keep its head above the body line on ventral suspension
C Fixate on an object at 15–20 cm
D Perform mouthing
E Turn towards the mother's voice

Question 45

Characteristic milestones in a 9-month-old infant are

A Points to small objects with index finger
B Arms extended in supine position
C Sits unsupported
D Shouts for attention
E Stands using furniture

Question 46

Developmental achievements in an 18-month-old child include

A Walks up and down stairs without help
B Speaks 2–3 recognisable words
C Enjoys simple pictures
D Scribbles
E Closes fist

Question 47

Children at the age of 2½ years will be able to

A Cut with scissors
B Stand on one foot momentarily
C Walk up stairs freely but use handrail to come down stairs
D Pull down pants and knickers at toilet
E Tie knots

Question 48

True or false?

A Smiling has usually started by the age of 6 months in most babies
B Walking in bottom shuffler babies has usually started at the age of 18–24 months
C Approximately 10% of children wet their beds at the age of 5–7 years
D Children are likely to start joining words at 3½ years old
E Children can ride a two-wheel bike without stabilisers at 6 years

Question 49

Delayed speech is mostly

A Due to psychogenic causes
B Due to mental retardation
C Due to tongue tie
D Familial
E Due to recurrent otitis media

Question 50

Inability to read may be due to

A Emotional factors
B Insecurity
C Poor environment
D Developmental delay
E Dyslexia

Question 51

Are the following statements about puberty true or false?

A Before puberty gonadotrophins are low because of positive feedback of gonadal sex hormones on the hypothalamus

B FSH is predominantly secreted by the pituitary

C Continual GnRH release is necessary for gonadotrophin secretion

D FSH is the first hormone to be secreted by both sexes

E LH is secreted mainly at night throughout puberty

Question 52

Are the following statements about staging of puberty true or false?

A Stage 2 genital development in boys is characterised by enlargement of the scrotum and testes without enlargement of the penis

B Stage 3 pubic hair in both sexes is characterised by slightly pigmented hair straight at the base of penis or along the labia

C Stage 4 breast development in girls is characterised by projection of papilla

D Stage 2 axillary hair in both sexes is characterised by scanty growth with slightly pigmented hair

E After the menarche only 3–5 cm of growth remain

Question 53

Common causes of pseudo-precocious puberty in girls rather than boys include

A Congenital adrenal hyperplasia

B Virilising adrenal tumour

C Hepatoblastoma

D Malignant embryonic tumour

E Functional follicular cyst

Question 54

Are the following statements about short stature in children true or false?

A Defined as height below the 3rd centile of weight

B Those with constitutional short stature will achieve normal height later

C In familial short stature, bone age is not consistent with chronological age

D Height velocity over a period of 4 months is important in predicting short stature

E Children more than 3 standard deviations below the mean almost always have a pathological cause for short stature

Question 55

True or false?

A Familial short stature is likely if the child's corrected height is above the 3rd centile

B Bone age is delayed in constitutional short stature and normal height velocity

C The commonest diagnostic cause of short stature in girls is Turner's syndrome

D Arrested growth with previous normal growth is common in chronic illness

E Hypopituitarism usually presents as a short newborn baby

Emergencies and resuscitation questions

Question 56

Atropine can be used

A In bradycardia accompanied by intubation
B If heart rate is less than 60 per minute with normal blood pressure and poor perfusion
C As a minimum dose of 0.1 mg but is not recommended in children
D But may be followed by meiosis
E To block vagal induced bradycardia.

Question 57

The most common causes of shock in children are

A Hypovolaemia
B Diabetic ketoacidosis
C Trauma
D Arrhythmias
E Heat

Question 58

Are the following statements about volume expansion true or false?

A Crystalloid solutions stay longer than colloids in the intravascular compartment
B Colloids are the ideal fluid replacement in paediatric trauma
C Dextrose-containing solution is ideal first-line fluid replacement in a shocked child
D 20 ml/kg should be given in cardiac arrest
E Decompensated shocked patients need more than 40 ml/kg of crystalloid fluid

Question 59

The alpha adrenergic effects of adrenaline

A Elevate the systolic blood pressure
B Increase renal blood flow
C Increase myocardial contractility
D Relax bronchial muscle
E Enhance delivery of oxygen to the heart

Question 60

Are the following statements about adrenaline true or false?

A Adrenaline can be used in treatment of symptomatic bradycardia (<60) in children
B May cause hypotension
C Not recommended in newborn babies with heart rate 60 and saturation 100% oxygen
D Can be infused using the same line as bicarbonate
E Action can be depressed by acidosis

Question 61

Are the following statements about adrenaline true or false?

A Cannot be given via ETT in neonates
B The first dose in children with cardiac arrest is 10 μg/kg of 1:10 000
C The second dose in neonates should be 100 μg/kg of 1:1000
D The peak level of adrenaline given via ETT is similar to IV
E Not recommended to be used as an infusion in children

Question 62

Are the following statements about acidosis true or false?

A May be due to accumulation of lactic acid in hypoxia
B Can follow hypercarbia
C Pa_{O_2} is important for correcting acidosis
D Can be corrected by hyperventilation in respiratory acidosis
E Vasoactive support will not help the correction of acidosis

Question 63

Are the following statements about bicarbonate true or false?

A Bicarbonate will not change the CSF pH
B It may cause change of intracellular pH
C It cannot be given via UVC
D It can be given via IO
E It can improve the survival rate in cardiac arrest if given early

Question 64

Bicarbonate may cause

A Shift of oxygen dissociation curve to the left
B Hyperkalaemia
C Hypocalcaemia
D Increased fibrillation threshold
E Hypernatraemia

Question 65

Prostaglandin can be used to keep the ductus open in the following conditions

A Moderate aortic stenosis
B Transposition of the great arteries
C Tricuspid atresia
D Persistent foetal circulation
E Coarctation of aorta

Question 66

Dopamine in low dosages

A Can cause increased renal blood flow
B Can cause increased coronary blood flow
C Can cause peripheral vessel bed dilatation
D Can cause increased noradrenaline secretion
E Is not effective in premature babies

Question 67

Are the following statements about dobutamine true or false?

A Acts on beta receptors
B Does not affect the splanchnic blood flow
C Increases cardiac output
D Decreases pulmonary capillary pressure
E Decreases systemic vascular resistance

Question 68

Lignocaine can be used in

A Ventricular tachycardia
B Ventricular fibrillation
C Status epilepticus
D Ventricular ectopics
E Supraventricular tachycardia

Question 69

Are the following statements about the ECG true or false?

A Depolarisation begins in the sino-atrial node
B A-V conductive tissue slows the electrical depolarisation
C The bundle of His depolarises the right ventricle
D The P wave represents the two atria
E Repolarisation is represented by the ST and T waves

Question 70

True or false?

A Cardiac output = stroke volume × heart rate
B Synchronised cardioversion is effective in tachyarrhythmias
C Slow arrhythmias are mainly due to congenital heart disease
D Absence of pulses may be associated with EMD
E Hypothyroidism may produce a flat ECG

Question 71

The following are the main causes of cardiac arrest in children

A Hypovolaemia
B Congenital heart disease
C Hypoxia
D Asthma
E Hypothermia

Question 72

True or false?

A A cuffed ETT can be used only after the age of 10 years
B Allowing an air leak in an uncuffed ETT is not appropriate for a ventilated child
C The cricoid membrane is between the thyroid cartilage and the cricoid cartilage
D A straight paddle laryngoscope cannot be used under the age of 1 year
E Chest thrust is not applicable for children below the age of 1 year

Immunology and allergy questions

Question 73

Are the following statements about cell-mediated immunity true or false?

A It activates the complement system
B Antigen-specific function is the role of the T-lymphocyte
C It is responsible for the delayed hypersensitivity reaction
D It activates T-cell mediators as it is important for cellular immunity
E Gamma interferon is an important mediator of B-cell activation

Question 74

The immune system in children is characterised by

A Interleukin 1 (IL-1) activates T cells to produce interleukin-2 (IL-2)
B Phagocytosis is performed mainly by polymorphonuclear leukocytes
C The alternative complement pathway uses factors C1–9
D IgG crosses the placenta
E The thymus gland is responsible for humoral immunity

Question 75

Wiskott–Aldrich syndrome is

A Autosomal dominant
B Associated with eczema
C Characterised by low lymphocyte count
D Associated with elevated IgA levels
E Associated with thrombocytosis

Question 76

Burton's syndrome

A Repeated ear infection is common
B It is inherited as X-linked autosomal recessive
C May be associated with arthritis
D Increases incidence of malignant diseases
E Intravenous immunoglobulin is usually required at 6–8 weekly intervals

Question 77

Chronic granulomatous disease in children is characterised by

A Autosomal dominant inheritance
B An abnormal oxidative metabolic response during phagocytosis
C Catalase-positive organisms as the main cause of recurrent infection
D Reduction in microbicidal activity
E Lack of cytochromes

Question 78

Leukocyte adhesion deficiency is

A Associated with delayed separation of umbilical cord
B Associated with osteomyelitis
C Associated with abnormal chemotaxis
D Due to lack of beta-chain (CD18)
E Associated with albinism

Question 79

Are the following statements about severe combined immune deficiency syndrome true or false?

A Usually inherited as X-linked recessive
B Prenatal diagnosis is possible in more than 20% of cases
C May be associated with low T-cell but normal B-cell counts
D BMT is not possible
E There is a functional defect in cell-mediated immunity and antibody production

Question 80

In ataxia telangiectasia

A Cerebellar ataxia is progressive
B There is impairment of cell-mediated immunity and antibody production
C There is a structural defect in a gene
D There is an association with malignant disease
E Granuloma formation is common

Question 81

Tests which can be done for cellular immunity include

A Nitroblue tetrazolium test
B Anti-B isohaemagglutinins
C Quantitative serum immunoglobulins
D CD4 and CD8
E Neutrophil motility

Question 82

Complement deficiency

A May be secondary to other diseases
B Is associated with defects in both classical and alternative pathways
C Of C1, C4 or C2 may present as lupus-like syndrome
D Of properdin may be associated with recurrent neisserial infection
E Of C3 may lead to hereditary angio-oedema

Question 83

Secondary immune deficiency

A Is associated with decreased production of immune components
B Is secondary to hypoproteinaemia
C Is associated with Hodgkin's lymphoma
D Sometimes requires Ig replacement
E Is not associated with drug therapy

Question 84

Acquired immune deficiency syndrome

A Is caused by retroviruses type 1 and 3
B Virus can be transmitted by close contact
C Is associated with persistent generalised lymphadenopathy
D Is associated with Kaposi's sarcoma
E May present as Cryptosporidium infection

Question 85

Major abnormalities associated with AIDS are

A Absolute depletion of CD8 lymphocytes
B Impaired delayed cutaneous hypersensitivity reactions
C Decreased interleukin-2 production
D Increased interferon-gamma production in response to antigens
E Persistent lymphopenia

Question 86

The following tests are useful in diagnosing HIV infection

A Antibodies by enzyme-linked immunoadsorbent assay (ELISA)
B Polymerase chain reaction (PCR)
C Immunoglobulin assay
D CD2:CD8 ratio
E White cell count

Question 87

Chemicals involved in allergic reactions and their mechanisms

A Histamine—increases cAMP
B Heparin—augments inactivation of prostaglandins
C Platelet-activating factor—leukocyte activation
D Prostaglandin-2—vasodilatation
E Thromboxane—leukocyte activation

Question 88

Are the following statements about allergy in children true or false?

A The late phase of a type I hypersensitivity reaction occurs at 8–12 hours
B Nasal mucosa may be blue in children
C The complement system is not involved
D Serotonin induces contraction of smooth muscle
E Type II reactions are mediated by IgE

Question 89

Non-allergic diseases associated with eosinophilia and high IgE include

A Hodgkin's disease
B Schistosomiasis
C DiGeorge anomaly
D Liver disease
E Thymic aplasia

Question 90

Skin tests in allergy

A A positive intradermal reaction is a weal of at least 15 mm induration
B A late phase reaction may occur if the weal exceeds 10 mm in diameter
C Oedema and erythema may last for 24 hours
D An immediate weal and flare indicates that the patient will experience clinical symptoms when exposed to the allergen
E Corticosteroids given for a few days prior to testing may lead to false negative results

Question 91

The Rast test

  A Is affected by antihistamines
  B Contains a broad selection of antigens
  C Is expensive
  D Carries a risk of allergic reaction
  E Is semiquantitative

Question 92

The following can be used as treatment in allergy or allergic reaction

  A Hyposensitisation
  B Adrenergics
  C Steroids
  D Adrenaline
  E Immunoglobulins

Question 93

Are the following statements about the ECG in children true or false?

A The T wave is usually opposite to the polarity of the QRS complex
B P waves are occasionally observed in asystole
C In VF, the P wave is identifiable
D In SVT the heart rate is usually below 220/minute
E Organised electrical activity is mainly associated with VF

Question 94

WPW syndrome

A Is associated with supraventricular tachycardia
B SVT responds very well to IV digoxin
C The majority of WPW syndromes are associated with cardiac structural abnormalities
D In Type A the accessory pathway is from right atrium to right ventricle
E May be associated with Ebstein's anomaly

Question 95

Features of ventricular septal defect include

A The commonest congenital heart anomalies, with an incidence of 40% in childhood
B Of small VSD, 80% will close before the age of 1 year
C The majority of VSD are medium sized
D Heart failure associated with large VSD often responds successfully to medication
E Prophylactic antibiotics are not recommended in small VSD prior to dental surgery

Question 96

Recognised features of ASD include

A Diastolic murmur at the right third intercostal space
B Association with Ellis–van Creveld syndrome
C Eisenmenger syndrome can follow untreated ASD
D ECG in ostium premium ASD is characterised by LAD and RBBB
E Delayed closure of pulmonary valve produces splitting of second heart sound which varies with respiration

Question 97

Patent ductus arteriosus is characterised by

A Blood flow through the duct from pulmonary to aortic arch during intrauterine life
B Machinery murmur can be heard on back as well as on front of chest
C Pulses are typically collapsed "water hammer"
D Pulse pressure is reduced and varies with respiration
E Anatomic closure of PDA occurs in the first week of life

Question 98

Characteristic features of coarctation of aorta include

A Blood pressure is higher in the upper limbs than the lower limbs
B Delayed femoral pulses
C Ejection systolic murmur on the second left intercostal space radiating to the neck and back
D Loud first heart sound
E Bilateral ventricular hypertrophy on ECG

Question 99

Are the following statements about Tetralogy of Fallot true or false?

A Systolic murmur is due to flow through VSD
B Soft second heart sound is due to early closure of aortic valve
C Squatting decreases the venous return to the heart, and lower pulmonary resistance
D Total correction is not possible during the first year of life
E Morphine and propranolol are used to prevent the hypoxic attacks

Question 100

In pulmonary stenosis

A Incidence is 8% of congenital heart diseases
B Balloon septostomy can be used as a palliative procedure for severe pulmonary stenosis
C Ejection click can be heard in infundibular stenosis
D The commonest lesion associated with Williams' syndrome
E Pulmonary vascular resistance increases without symptoms

Question 101

Transposition of the great arteries is characterised by

A Cyanosis in the early hours after delivery
B Pansystolic murmur on the right third intercostal space
C Single second heart sound
D Pulmonary artery trunk lying in front of the aortic arch
E Normal heart size on the CXR in early days of life

Question 102

In Ebstein's anomaly

A The tricuspid annulus is displaced into the left ventricle
B There is an association with tall P wave on ECG
C Fast heart beat and cyanosis are the early signs
D Cyanosis becomes worse with time as the pulmonary vascular resistance increases
E There may be an association with WPW syndrome

Question 103

Early signs of heart failure in infants include

A Oedema
B Sweating
C Hepatomegaly
D Raised JVP
E Tachycardia

Question 104

Prophylactic antibiotics are indicated in

A ASD
B VSD
C Coarctation of aorta
D Dilated cardiomyopathy
E Coronary artery aneurysm

Question 105

Are the following statements about heart failure in children true or false?

A Fluid restriction is necessary
B Nasogastric tube feeding is not needed in babies
C Digoxin is the first drug of choice
D Congenital heart diseases are the most common cause
E Hyperkalaemia may follow treatment of heart failure with diuretics

Question 106

Major factors that lead to a decrease in rheumatic fever incidence include

A Improvements in hygiene in the community
B Improvement in social classes
C Early diagnosis
D Vaccination against streptococci and other bacteria
E Prevention of recurrence

Question 107

Early manifestations of bacterial endocarditis include

A Pyrexia of unknown origin
B Thrombo-embolic phenomena
C Anaemia
D Haematuria
E Splenomegaly

Question 108

Are the following statements about hypertension in children and its associations true or false?

A High renin level and hypernatraemia are associated with Conn's disease
B If diastolic pressure is less than 100 in the 13–18 year age group, there is no need to investigate
C Diuretics are used as the first line of treatment in acute hypertension
D Intravenous diazoxide may lead to hypoglycaemia
E Atenolol is more effective in acute cases of high BP

Question 109

Are the following statements about pericarditis true or false?

A A friction rub is present in >50% of all cases
B There is an inverted ST wave segment on ECG
C There is always pericardial fluid on echocardiography
D There is a flattened T wave on ECG
E There are changes in the quality of the murmur

Question 110

Beta-blockers

A Reduce the high BP by vasodilatation
B Cause nightmares
C Can cause hypoglycaemia
D Can be used in thyrotoxicosis
E Can be used in heart failure

Question 111

Arterial dilatation can be caused by

A Increase in P_{CO_2}
B Increase in P_{O_2}
C Propranolol
D Histamine
E Aldosterone

Question 112

In ECG

A P–R interval <0.12 seconds is normal
B Frontal plane of QRS axis lying between −30 and +90 is abnormal
C In left ventricular failure the sum of S wave in V6 plus R wave in V1 is >35 mm
D Broad and notched P wave is indicative of left atrial enlargement
E U wave in hypokalaemia

Question 113

Pulmonary stenosis rather than atrial septal defect can be diagnosed if there is

A RBBB on ECG
B Parasternal heave
C Fixed splitting of second heart sound
D Early ejection click at the apex
E Right ventricular hypertrophy

Question 114

In cardiac dysrhythmias

A Permanent pacemaker is needed for acquired complete heart block
B Exacerbation of ventricular tachycardia during exercise does not need further investigation
C Prolongation of Q–T on ECG during exercise is normal
D Complete heart block is usually congenital
E SLE can cause a conduction defect in babies

Question 115

Common cardiac abnormalities associated with syndromes are

A Down's syndrome—AVSD
B Marfan's syndrome—coarctation of aorta
C Williams' syndrome—subvalvular aortic stenosis
D Holt–Oram syndrome—arrhythmias
E Ellis–van Creveld syndrome—ASD

Question 116

Cardiac abnormalities associated with the following conditions include

A Pompe's disease—cardiomyopathy
B Friedreich's ataxia—coronary artery dilatation
C Muscular dystrophy—myocardial degeneration
D Hyperlipoproteinaemia—atherosclerosis
E Maple syrup urine disease—cardiomyopathy

Respiratory questions

Question 117

Are the following statements about cardiovascular-pulmonary changes in newborn babies true or false?

A Increase in systemic vascular resistance
B Decrease in pulmonary vascular resistance
C Physiological closure of PDA and foramen ovale in the first few days of life
D Continuing manufacture of surfactant even outside the uterus
E Peripheral and central chemoreceptors are not immediately active because they lack maturity

Question 118

Hyperventilation may occur in

A Salicylate overdose
B Guillain–Barré syndrome
C Obesity
D Diabetes mellitus
E Renal failure

Question 119

Which of the following are useful in assessing the severity of an asthma attack in children?

A Pulse rate
B Peak expiratory flow rate
C P_{CO_2}
D Use of accessory muscles
E Respiratory rate

Question 120

Are the following statements about the respiratory system true or false?

A The lungs contain small muscles which help in breathing
B Expiration is an active process during quiet breathing
C The P_{O_2} in the arterial blood is influenced by the P_{O_2} of the venous blood
D The lungs can produce hormones, e.g. angiotensin II, prostacyclines
E The P_{CO_2} is directly proportional to alveolar ventilation

Question 121

Cyanosis can occur with

A ≥5 g/l of deoxygenated haemoglobin in blood
B Polycythaemia
C Methaemoglobinaemia
D Anaemia
E Lung diseases

Question 122

Respiratory failure is associated with

A Mechanical abnormalities of lungs and chest wall
B Chronic rather than acute pulmonary disease
C Cyanosis
D Hypocapnia
E Stress ulcers

Question 123

Crackles are heard in the following conditions

A Foreign body inhalation
B Lung abscess
C Pulmonary oedema
D Cystic fibrosis
E Atypical pneumonia

Question 124

Erythema nodosum

A Lesions are painful
B Lesions occur only below the knees
C May occur in infective endocarditis
D Is a type IV immune reaction
E Often follows a virus infection

Question 125

Cheyne–Stokes respiration

A Is characterised by rapid and slow respiration with pauses of apnoea
B May occur in normal people
C Usually follows severe head injuries
D Occurs in both types of respiratory failure, types I and II
E Mostly responds to oxygen therapy

Question 126

The manifestations of pneumothorax in children are

A Chest pain
B Exertional dyspnoea
C Shift of mediastinum to the affected side
D Haemoptysis
E Normal pulse

Question 127

Compensated respiratory acidosis

A pH is low
B Bicarbonate is low
C P_{CO_2} is high
D P_{O_2} is normal
E May occur in cystic fibrosis

Question 128

Features that may be associated with cystic fibrosis on first presentation are

A Oedema of the feet
B Anaemia
C Nasal polyps
D Rectal prolapse
E Hyperpigmented skin patches

Question 129

Complications associated with cystic fibrosis include

A Cor pulmonale
B Liver cancer
C Equivalent intussusception
D Hypertrophic osteoarthropathy
E Insulin-dependent diabetes mellitus

Question 130

Side effects of drugs used to treat pulmonary tuberculosis are as follows

A Tetracycline—cataract
B Isoniazid—peripheral neuropathy
C Ethambutol—macrocytic anaemia
D Pyrazinamide—discoloration of teeth
E Dapsone—loss of hair

Question 131

Recognised causes of a transudate pleural effusion are

A Rheumatoid arthritis
B Malignancy
C Lymphangiectasia
D Heart failure
E Nephrotic syndrome

Question 132

Points in favour of epiglottitis rather than croup are

A Inspiratory croup
B Barking cough
C Toxic status
D Rapid deterioration
E Respiratory failure

Question 133

Recognised causes of chronic cough in children include

A Hiatus hernia
B Foreign body
C Exposure to irritant
D Mycoplasma infection
E Smoking

Question 134

Primary pulmonary hypertension is characterised by

A Variable response to O_2 therapy
B High pulmonary vascular resistance after birth as a cause
C Polycythaemia as a cause
D Abnormal ECG
E Persistent foetal circulation as the commonest cause

Question 135

In cystic fibrosis

A Infertility is more common in males
B Biliary cirrhosis becomes symptomatic in only 10–15% of patients
C The delta 508 deletion is the commonest mutation
D One third of patients present with meconium ileus
E Incidence is 1:20 000 of population worldwide

Question 136

In RSV-positive bronchiolitis

A Two thirds will have recurrent wheeze within the first year after infection

B Fine expiratory crackles are characteristic

C Use of IM monoclonal antibodies reduces the frequency of admissions in premature babies with chronic lung diseases

D Bronchodilators are the major symptom relief

E Inhaled steroids shorten the length of admission

Gastroenterology questions

Question 137

Motility of the alimentary tract is characterised by

A The alimentary tract is composed of smooth muscle
B Peristaltic waves relax the oesophageal sphincter
C Tonic contraction of the stomach is stimulated by the arrival of food
D Colonic propulsion consists of contraction rings forming and disappearing over long periods, leading to elimination of faeces
E Segmentation is the main activity of the colon and increases in constipation

Question 138

Are the following statements about fat metabolism true or false?

A It predominantly occurs in the duodenum and upper jejunum
B Dietary fat occurs in the form of triglycerides which are hydrolysed by pancreatic lipase to fatty acids and lipoproteins
C Micelles contain fatty acids, monoglycerides and bile acids
D Absorption of long chain fatty acids occurs in the re-esterified form of triglycerides
E Lipoproteins and chylomicrons are transported to the venous circulation

Question 139

The following are common causes of dysphagia

A Achalasia
B Tonsillitis
C Parotitis
D Oesophageal atresia
E Myasthenia gravis

Question 140

The following conditions predispose to gastro-oesophageal reflux

A Repair of pyloric stenosis
B Hiatus hernia
C Repair of diaphragmatic hernia
D Cerebral palsy
E Pernicious anaemia

Question 141

Aphthous ulceration of the mouth can be associated with

A Crohn's disease
B Renal failure
C Gluten sensitivity enteropathy
D Chicken pox
E Gastric ulcer

Question 142

Pyloric stenosis

A Is more common in males
B Commonly presents in the first 3 months of life
C Projectile vomiting occurs I hour after a feed
D May be associated with diarrhoea
E Abdominal peristalsis from left to right is a diagnostic feature

Question 143

The most common causes of vomiting in infancy are

A Pyloric stenosis
B Adrenal hyperplasia syndrome
C Gastro-oesophageal reflux
D Cow's milk protein intolerance
E Infection

Question 144

Common causes of malabsorption in children are

A Toddler diarrhoea
B Lymphoma
C Food hypersensitivity
D Cow's milk protein intolerance
E Giardiasis

Question 145

Failure to thrive is commonly associated with

A Congenital heart diseases
B Asthma
C Bronchiectasis
D Diabetes mellitus
E Obstructive sleep apnoea

Question 146

Recurrent abdominal pain in children is mostly due to

A Constipation
B Food allergy
C Psychological stress
D Abdominal migraine
E Thread worms

Question 147

Appendicitis in children can be associated with

A Frequent vomiting
B Abnormal urine analysis
C Temperature of 39–40C° with flushing
D Diarrhoea
E Periumbilical tenderness

Question 148

Common features of coeliac disease are

A Anorexia
B Very smelly, pale and bulky stool
C Failure to thrive from birth
D Wasted buttocks with short stature
E Abdominal distension with palpable liver

Question 149

Intussusception may be associated with the following

A Cystic fibrosis
B Hirschsprung's disease
C Henoch–Schönlein purpura
D Gastroenteritis
E Rectal prolapse

Question 150

Histopathological findings supporting a diagnosis of Crohn's disease rather than ulcerative colitis are

A Crypt abscesses, haemorrhage and ulceration
B Non-caseating granulomas
C Lead-pipe appearance
D Shortening of the intestine
E Transmural inflammation

Question 151

Features of upper intestinal obstruction are

A Intermittent pain
B Constipation
C Absence of gases in the lower abdomen by AXR
D Increased intestinal motility
E Bilious vomiting

Question 152

Are the following statements about liver function true or false?

A Gluconeogenesis uses amino acids from peripheral tissues to maintain blood glucose and to produce glycogen
B The majority of proteins involved in clot formation are produced by the liver
C Albumin is the first protein to be produced during foetal life
D In severe liver damage, the serum level of branched amino acids is increased
E Cholesterol is the precursor of bile acids

Question 153

True or false?

A More than 90% of bilirubin synthesis is from HbA haemoglobin in the newborn
B More than 80% of bilirubin is in conjugated form
C Acidosis and drugs may cause kernicterus at a low level of bilirubin
D UDPG-transferase plays a role in transport of bilirubin
E Cholic and chenodeoxycholic acids are secondary bile acids

Question 154

Causes of unconjugated hyperbilirubinaemia in infants and children include

A Dubin–Johnson and Rotor syndrome
B Novobiocin
C Viral hepatitis
D Sickle cell anaemia
E Hypothyroidism

Question 155

Are the following statements about Reye's syndrome true or false?

A Hyperammonaemia is diagnostic
B The objective to be achieved is treatment of the cerebral oedema
C The major site of injury is the mitochondria
D It is not associated with chicken pox
E The gross pathological feature in the liver is fatty change

Question 156

Phenomena associated with chronic active hepatitis are

A Pericarditis
B Nephritis
C Thyroiditis
D Fibrosing alveolitis
E Cushing's syndrome

Question 157

True or false?

A Corticosteroids have proved to be effective in treatment of negative HbsAg.
B One third of children with chronic active hepatitis progress to liver cirrhosis despite treatment
C The pathological changes in chronic active hepatitis are perilobular hepatitis and piecemeal erosion to parenchyma
D Chronic persistent hepatitis leads to cirrhosis
E There is an association between liver fibrosis and polycystic kidney disease in children

Question 158

Are the following statements about Wilson's disease true or false?

A Caeruloplasmin is low
B It can present with dementia during adolescence
C Increased amounts of copper in liver biopsy are diagnostic
D It can be treated with zinc
E An increase in urinary copper is a sign of improvement after therapy

Question 159

Common features of portal hypertension include

A Ascites
B Protein losing enteropathy
C Diarrhoea
D Oesophageal varices
E Cutaneous porto-systemic shunt

Question 160

In ascites

A Hypoalbuminaemia reduces osmotic pressure and hydrostatic pressure within the vessels.
B Hypoalbuminaemia leads to more fluid entering the hepatic venous system
C Fluid retention decreases water absorption by the kidneys
D Fluid retention increases renin secretion
E Initial presentation may be with a hernia

Question 161

Genetic causes of cirrhosis include

A Fructosaemia
B Chronic active hepatitis
C Cystinosis
D Thalassaemia
E Zellweger's syndrome

Metabolic disorder questions

Question 162

In insulin-dependent diabetes mellitus (IDDM)

A Absolute lack of insulin differentiates it from adult onset DM
B Children are usually obese
C There is an association with HLA-B8
D Children can present with failure to thrive
E Detection of glycosuria is diagnostic

Question 163

True or false?

A The Somogyi effect is due to bouts of hypoglycaemia followed by hyperglycaemia
B Glycosuria and ketonuria with high insulin therapy are features of the Somogyi effect
C The association between primary autoimmune hypothyroidism and IDDM in the general population is low
D Diabetic dwarfism is associated with hepatomegaly
E Insulin requirements during infection in a patient with IDDM can be increased by 50%

Question 164

In hypoinsulinaemia

A Ketones will be high due to complete utilisation of fat
B Decreased glucose clearance leads to loss of water and electrolytes
C Dehydration impairs renal function, with low P_{CO_2} and low bicarbonate in lungs
D Blood glucose is always high
E The incidence of thrombosis is increased

Question 165

Criteria for DKA are

A Leukocytosis is common
B 15% dehydration
C Serum osmolality is high
D Hyperventilation and ketosis are indicative of acidosis
E Positive clintest of glucose >20 mmol/l is diagnostic

Question 166

In treatment of DKA

A Normal saline (0.9% NaCl) is the only fluid that can be used as first replacement fluid
B A loading IV insulin dose is to be given immediately
C Insulin pump infusion with short-acting insulin is the current therapy
D Subcutaneous insulin therapy can be used as a substitute for infusion
E NaHCO$_3$ must be given if pH is less than 7.2

Question 167

Recognised long-term sequelae after prolonged hypoglycaemia in infants are

A Mental retardation
B Recurrent seizures
C Personality problems
D Infertility
E Hydrocephalus

Question 168

Drugs that can be used in treatment of hyperinsulinaemia include

A Chlorothiazides
B Propranolol
C Glucagon
D Diazoxide
E Chlorpropamide

Question 169

Are the following associations between disorders and enzyme defects true or false?

A Von Gierke's disease—galactose-1-phosphate uridyl transferase deficiency
B Phenylketonuria—phenylalanine reductase
C Urea cycle defect—ornithine transamine carboxylase deficiency
D Lesch–Nyhan syndrome—purine nucleoside phosphorylase deficiency
E Gaucher's disease—hexoaminadase B

Question 170

Are the following statements about the inheritance of each disease true or false?

A Marfan's syndrome—autosomal dominant
B Hurler's syndrome—autosomal recessive
C Hunter's syndrome—X-linked dominant
D Cystinosis—autosomal dominant
E Tyrosinaemia—autosomal recessive

Question 171

Clinical features of glycogen storage disease type Ia include

A Hyperlipidaemia
B Convulsions with hepatosplenomegaly
C Neutropenia and thrombocytopenia
D Enlarged kidneys
E Muscle weakness after exercise

Question 172

Beta oxidation defect is characterised by

A Hypoketonaemia
B Hyperinsulinaemia
C Hypertriglyceridaemia
D MCAD (medium chain acyl-CoA-dehydrogenase deficiency) being the commonest form
E Association with cot death

Question 173

In fructosaemia

A The cause is fructose 1,6 phosphate aldolase deficiency
B Hyperventilation is common
C A fructose tolerance test is indicated to measure response to hypoglycaemia
D Presentation is usually later than that of other carbohydrate metabolism defects
E Hyperammonaemia is uncommon

Question 174

Hyperlipidaemia in children

A Hyperchylomicronaemia is inherited as autosomal recessive
B Type II is familial and there is no autosomal inheritance
C Familial hypercholesterolaemia is inherited as autosomal dominant.
D Familial hypercholesterolaemia is associated with heart disease
E Hyperlipoproteinaemia is associated with high cholesterol

Question 175

In porphyria

A There is a defect in the heme biosynthetic pathway
B Acute intermittent porphyria may present with muscle pain and vomiting
C Congenital erythropoietic porphyria is associated with early presentation with hypersensitivity
D Pink urine in infancy may be due to porphyria cutanea tarda
E Neurological symptoms are commonly associated with hereditary coproporphyria

Question 176

Ketotic hyperglycinaemia

A Usually presents after the first birthday
B Is associated with myoclonic seizures as the initial presentation
C Is associated with high glycine concentration in CSF
D Sodium valproate reduces the plasma glycine level
E Is associated with a defect in p protein

Endocrinology questions

Question 177

In the hypothalamus

A The neurosecretory cells are osmoreceptors and volume receptors
B Oxytocin and vasopressin are the only neurohumoral substances in hypothalamic nuclei
C DDAVP is secreted by the hypothalamus
D Oxytocin is responsible for uterine contraction.
E Vasopressin pressor effects are obtained by physiological rather than pharmacological quantities in the hypothalamus

Question 178

Likely common causes of diabetes insipidus include

A Tuberculoma
B Brain tumours
C Leukaemia
D Idiopathic
E Trauma

Question 179

True or false?

A Urine osmolality remains low in nephrogenic DI after a vasopressin test
B Total daily sodium excretion in urine is increased in central DI
C Urine osmolality is <200 mOsm/kg of water in both CDI and NDI
D Urine osmolality is >280 mOsm/kg of water in psychogenic polydipsia after a water deprivation test
E Synthetic arginine-vasopressin (DDAVP) is effective orally in CDI

Question 180

Metabolic actions of growth hormone

A Decreases glucose uptake by muscle
B Can decrease plasma alpha amino acid
C May cause rise in blood glucose
D Has a diabetogenic action
E Increases adipose tissue lipids

Question 181

Cushing's syndrome is characterised by

A Short stature
B Hypertension
C Pale skin
D Osteoporosis
E Hypokalaemia

Question 182

Known causes of growth hormone deficiency include

A Developmental midline defect
B Anti-leukaemia therapy
C Autoimmune diseases
D TB meningitis
E Waterhouse–Friedrichsen syndrome

Question 183

Obesity is mostly associated with the following conditions or syndromes

A Laurence–Moon–Biedl syndrome
B Hyperpituitarism
C Fröhlich's tumour
D Addison's disease
E Prader–Willi syndrome

Question 184

Recognised features associated with congenital adrenal hyperplasia (CAH-21) are

A Vomiting
B Diarrhoea
C Hyperkalaemia
D High blood pressure
E High urinary sodium chloride

Question 185

The salt-losing variant of adrenogenital syndrome occurs with the following enzyme deficiencies

A 20,22-desmolase deficiency
B Congenital adrenal hypoplasia
C 17α-hydroxylase deficiency
D Females with 21-hydroxylase deficiency
E 11β-hydroxylase deficiency

Question 186

True or false?

A 17α-hydroxyprogesterone is high in 21-hydroxylase deficiency
B IV steroids are the first emergency treatment in salt-losing CAH
C Fluids used to treat salt-losing CAH must be hypertonic with dextrose
D Tall stature is the end result in children with CAH due to 21-hydroxylase deficiency
E Precocious puberty occurs only in males with 21-hydroxylase deficiency

Question 187

Recognised side effects of glucocorticoids are

A Muscular weakness
B Amenorrhoea
C Peptic ulceration
D Hypercalcaemia
E Metabolic alkalosis

Question 188

Addison's disease is associated with

A Alopecia
B Insulin-dependent diabetes
C Pancreatic insufficiency
D Medullary carcinoma of thyroid
E Hyperparathyroidism

Question 189

In hypoaldosteronism

A The cause is hyperplasia of zona fasciculata and zona glomerulosa and adenoma.

B Nocturnal diuresis is frequently present

C Hypertension is uncommonly present

D Hypokalaemia is common

E Total adrenalectomy is required

Question 190

Are the following statements about the adrenal medulla true or false?

A Both adrenaline and noradrenaline are synthesised from tyrosine via DOPA to dopamine by decarboxylation

B More than 1 microgram of catecholamines is circulating in blood

C A third of catecholamines are secreted as vanillyl mandelic acid (VMA) in urine

D Homovanillic acid (HVA) is the metabolite of adrenaline

E Chromaffin cells are found only in the adrenal medulla

Question 191

In normal genitalia

A The primitive human gonad starts to develop between the sixth and eighth week of foetal life

B H-Y histocompatibility antigen is the initial determinant for the male phenotype

C Testosterone and anti-mullerian hormone start to be secreted by the testes from the eighth week of foetal life

D Leydig cells produce anti-mullerian hormone which inhibits mullerian duct development

E Virilisation of external genitalia is completed by binding of dihydrotestosterone to a cytoplasmic receptor between the 8th and 14th weeks of foetal life

Question 192

True or false?

A The iodotyrosines do not enter the blood and are used in coupling

B The iodotyrosines are used again for T3 and T4 synthesis

C Most T3 is secreted by the thyroid gland

D There is placental transfer of T3 and T4

E The active form of T3 and T4 is bound to TBG

Question 193

Clinical features of acquired hypothyroidism include

A Mental retardation
B Growth failure
C Dry, sparse hair
D Tibial myxoedema
E Slow reflex relaxation

Question 194

In Hashimoto's disease

A Inheritance is autosomal dominant
B Increase in anti-thyroid antibodies is diagnostic
C Serum T4 is low and serum T3 is normal in the euthyroid state
D There may be manifestations of hyperthyroidism
E Goitre can be reduced with thyroxine therapy

Question 195

Deficiency of parathyroid hormone is usually associated with the following

A Hypercalcaemia
B Hyperphosphataemia
C Diminished plasma 1,25(OH)2D
D Generalised convulsions
E High alkaline phosphatase

Haematology questions

Question 196

Reticulocytes are usually greater than 2% in

A Elliptocytosis
B Pure red cell aplasia
C Autoimmune haemolytic anaemia
D Vitamin B_{12} deficiency
E Glucose-6-phosphate dehydrogenase deficiency

Question 197

A leukaemoid reaction may be associated with

A Tuberculosis
B Leukoerythroblastic anaemia
C Intoxication
D Severe haemorrhage
E Whooping cough

Question 198

In von Willebrand's disease

A Platelet count is low
B PTT is prolonged
C Thrombin time is normal
D Factors vW-Ag and VIIIC are reduced
E Inherited as autosomal dominant

Question 199

Characteristic features of Fanconi anaemia are

A Exocrine pancreatic dysfunction
B Dystrophic nails
C Absent thumb
D GCSF is of more benefit as treatment than GMCSF
E Lymphopenia

Question 200

Are the following statements about Schwachmann syndrome true or false?

A GCSF is very effective in increasing neutrophil count
B Bone marrow transplant is not effective
C Corticosteroids give some haematological improvement
D Androgens are used as treatment
E Chlorothiazides can help to improve absorption

Question 201

Are the following statements about diseases and their associations true or false?

A Kostmann's syndrome—neutropenia
B Diamond–Blackfan syndrome—thrombocytopenia
C Paroxysmal nocturnal haemoglobinuria—thrombosis
D Parvovirus B19—pure red cell aplasia
E Sideroblastic anaemia—liver diseases

Question 202

The following tests are diagnostic for iron deficiency anaemia

A Serum ferritin
B Plasma iron and total iron binding capacity ratio
C Mean corpuscular haemoglobin concentration
D Mean corpuscular volume
E Radio immunoassay of plasma TFR

Question 203

Ring sideroblasts may be associated with poisoning by

A Mercury
B Zinc
C Copper
D Gold
E Lead

Question 204

Iron overload may occur with the following conditions

A β-Thalassaemia
B Sickle cell disease
C Chronic haemoglobinuria
D Zellweger's syndrome
E Hereditary tyrosinaemia

Question 205

Are the following statements about red cell indices in chronic diseases true or false?

A Mean corpuscular volume is normal
B Iron level is high
C Ferritin is high
D Mean corpuscular haemoglobin is low
E Total iron binding capacity is normal

Question 206

Parenteral iron therapy should always be avoided in the following

A Children
B Nephrotic syndrome
C Kwashiorkor
D Poor compliance with oral therapy
E Where parasites are endemic

Question 207

Characteristic features of pernicious anaemia include

A Association with autoimmune gastritis
B Association with achloryhydria
C Association with polyendocrinopathy syndrome
D Absent intrinsic factor production
E Sometimes follows ileal resection

Question 208

Folate deficiency may occur in

A Liver diseases
B Anti-convulsant therapy
C Gluten-induced enteropathy
D Ring worm infection
E Radiotherapy treatment

Question 209

Cold-reactive antibody haemolytic anaemia occurs in

A Systemic lupus erythematosus
B Post viral infection
C Epstein–Barr virus infection
D Quinine-induced anaemia
E Lymphoproliferative disorders

Question 210

Are the following statements about the Coombs test true or false?

A Weakly positive in ABO incompatibility
B It is an anti-globulin test
C Direct test will detect IgG
D Indirect test useful in alloimmune reaction
E May be used in room temperature

Question 211

Drugs that may cause autoimmune haemolytic anaemia include

A Methyldopa
B Frusemide
C Penicillin
D Sulphonamide
E Digoxin

Question 212

Clinical features associated with sickle cell disease include

A Acute splenic sequestration
B Chronic hypersplenism
C Renal stones
D Salmonella septicaemia
E Dactylitis

Question 213

A child presented with painful lower limbs and raised temperature. He is known to have HBSS. Are the following approaches to management correct or otherwise?

A IV fluids—normal maintenance
B IV antibiotics
C Exchange transfusion
D Lower limb X-ray
E Immediate IV morphine infusion

Question 214

Laboratory findings in haemolytic anaemia are

A Increased haptoglobin
B Reticulocytosis
C Heinz bodies
D Target cells
E Ghost cells

Question 215

In thalassaemia

A There is a reduction in globin chain synthesis
B Hypochromia is common
C There is a cell membrane defect
D 2–3% HbF is present
E The condition usually manifests soon after birth

Question 216

Anaemias associated with a red cell membrane defect are

A Pyruvate kinase deficiency
B Spherocytosis
C Thalassaemia
D Pyropoikilocytosis
E Abetalipoproteinaemia

Question 217

Target cells are commonly seen in these conditions

A Following splenectomy
B Iron deficiency anaemia
C Liver diseases
D Sickle cell disease
E Aplastic anaemia

Question 218

Neutropenia is associated with

A Fanconi anaemia
B Glycogen storage disease type Ia
C Sepsis
D Penicillinamine treatment
E Brucellosis

Question 219

Eosinophilia is associated with the following

A Giardiasis
B Gentamicin treatment
C Dermatitis herpetiformis
D Chicken pox
E Ulcerative colitis

Question 220

Conditions associated with an increased incidence of acute leukaemia include

A Bloom's syndrome
B Treatment with alkylating agents
C Viral infection
D Carbon monoxide intoxication
E Aplastic anaemia

Question 221

Thrombocytopenia with abnormally shaped platelets is commonly associated with

A Bernard–Soulier syndrome
B Wiskott–Aldrich syndrome
C TAR syndrome
D Immune deficiency
E Haemolytic syndrome

Nephrology questions

Question 222

Fluid requirements are increased in children with the following conditions

A Children and infants nursed in a humidified area
B Pyrexia
C Cystic fibrosis
D Pneumonia
E Thyrotoxicosis

Question 223

In hyponatraemia

A ECF is invariably reduced
B Oliguria is common
C The condition can be caused only by loss of sodium in excess of water
D Hypotonic enemas are a frequent cause
E Hyperlipidaemia can cause low Na level

Question 224

Oedema is usually due to

A Decrease in capillary blood pressure as in cardiac failure
B Decrease in colloidal oncotic pressure
C Milroy's disease
D Decrease in permeability of the capillaries
E Increase in capillary blood pressure in burns

Question 225

Are the following statements about the treatment of hypo-natraemia true or false?

A Diuretics only in cases associated with oedema with fluid overload
B Sodium deficit may be approximated as follows $(140 - \text{plasma Na}) \times 0.6 \times \text{body weight}$
C In renal failure by insensible losses plus any other losses from salt and water
D In chronic SIADH by demeclocycline
E In excessive water intake by diuretics

Question 226

Are the following statements about hypernatraemia and its therapy true or false?

A Convulsions can precede and follow treatment
B Iodogenic osmoles occur pre treatment and lead to brain haemorrhage
C Hypocalcaemia and hyperglycaemia frequently occur
D Fluid therapy in the form of 0.18% NaCl and 5% dextrose in the first 48 hours is commonly used
E Commonly follows treatment of intracranial hypertension

Question 227

In hypokalaemia

A One of the common causes is diuretic therapy
B ECG changes take the form of a high amplitude P wave and inverted T wave
C The maximum potassium infusion should be 0.50 mmol/kg/h
D Potassium chloride can be used in all hypokalaemic cases
E Smooth muscle only is affected

Question 228

The early presentation of post-streptococcal glomerulonephritis includes

A Dyspnoea
B Haematuria
C Swelling of scrotum and legs
D High blood pressure
E Red cell and glomerular casts in urine

Question 229

False positive results of proteinuria may occur in the following conditions

A Alkaline urine
B Gross haematuria
C Acid urine
D Metabolites of sulphonamides
E Non-albumin proteinuria

Question 230

Are the following statements about nephrotic syndrome true or false?

A More than 80% of patients with MPGN will have haematuria
B Hypertension is found in membranous nephropathy in more than 30% of patients
C Irrespective of morphology, 50% of children with NS respond completely to steroid therapy even when haematuria is present
D Nitrogen retention occurs in 20% of patients with FSGS
E C3 is low in MPGN

Question 231

Indications for renal biopsy include

A Any patient below one year of age with nephrotic syndrome
B Acute renal failure that has not responded to treatment for 2–3 weeks
C Chronic renal failure
D NS with normal C3 level
E Steroid-dependent disease

Question 232

Common causes of secondary infantile nephrotic syndrome include

A Renal vein thrombosis
B DRASH syndrome
C Syphilis
D Toxoplasmosis
E Idiopathic membranous glomerulopathy

Question 233

The main causes of haematuria in infants and children are

A Berger's disease
B Alport's syndrome
C Calculus
D Tumours
E Factitious

Question 234

Are the following statements about conditions and their associations with renal malformations true or false?

A Branchio-oto-renal syndrome—renal hypoplasia
B Prune belly syndrome—renal medullary dysplasia
C Tuberous sclerosis—hamartomas
D VATER association—renal aplasia in 50%
E Ehlers–Danlos syndrome—renal cysts

Question 235

Bilateral kidney enlargement is usually associated with

A Posterior urethral valve
B Ectopic kidney
C Renal artery stenosis
D Wilms' tumour
E Pelvi-ureteric junction obstruction

Question 236

Causes of dysuria include

A Balanitis
B Isoniazid
C Henoch–Schönlein purpura
D Wilms' tumour
E Bladder neck irritation by calculus

Question 237

Primary glomerulonephritis is associated with the following disorders

A Amyloidosis
B Immune complex glomerulonephritis (idiopathic)
C FSGS
D DM
E Shunt nephritis

Question 238

Methods used to treat hyperkalaemia in ARF to remove K from the body are

A IV 10% calcium gluconate
B Glucose + insulin
C Peritoneal dialysis
D IV 7.5% $NaHCO_3$
E Ion exchange resins

Question 239

Are the following associations between therapies and management of ARF true or false?

A Propranolol—hypertension
B 1000 ml insensible losses + urine output—replacement fluid over 24 hours
C Fluid restriction—hyponatraemia
D Aluminium hydroxide—hypocalcaemia
E 800 kcal/m^2 of body surface—nutrition

Question 240

Indications for dialysis in renal failure are

A High P waves on ECG
B Pericarditis and bleeding
C Urea serum level 15 mmol/l
D Fluid overload with hypertension
E Feeding problem

Question 241

Advantages of peritoneal dialysis over haemodialysis in children include

A Can be done in any hospital
B There is no risk of infection which occurs in haemodialysis
C Tolerated well by obese patients
D Quickly corrects biochemical states
E Is safe in a patient who will have abdominal surgery

Question 242

Laboratory findings in distal renal tubular acidosis are

A Hypercalciuria
B Hyperkalaemia
C Renal glycosuria
D Hypophosphataemia
E Generalised aminoaciduria

Question 243

Recognised causes of renal concentrating defect are

A Lithium
B Hyperkalaemia
C Sickle cell disease
D Mannitol
E Medullary cystic disease

Question 244

Known causes of pyuria that can lead to misdiagnosis of UTI are

A Renal tumour
B Fever
C Adenitis
D Malignancy
E Vulvovaginitis

Question 245

Conditions causing hypercalcaemia and hypercalciuria which lead to medullary nephrocalcinosis include

A Distal renal tubular acidosis
B Primary hyperparathyroidism
C Renal cortical necrosis
D Oxalosis
E Vitamin D toxicity

Neuroanatomy and neurophysiology questions

Question 246

Are the following associations between peripheral nerves and their origins true or false?

A Radial—C6,7
B Median—C6,7,8
C Femoral—S1,2
D Ulnar—C8,T1
E Musculocutaneous—C5,6

Question 247

True or false?

A The brachial plexus originates from C4,5,6,7,8 and T1
B The main branches of the lateral cord are the ulnar nerve and median nerve
C The long thoracic nerve originates from C5,6,7
D The radial nerve is the main branch of the posterior cord
E There are 12 intercostal nerves

Question 248

Are the following statements about the radial nerve true or false?

A Originates from lateral posterior and medial cord
B If injured may lead to wrist drop
C The superficial radial nerve supplies the extensor pollicis longus
D Supplies sensory area over the ring and little fingers
E Main supply for extensor muscle groups of upper limb

Question 249

Features of the lumbar plexus

A Its roots originate from T1,2,L1,2,3,4,5
B The lateral femoral cutaneous nerve arises from L2,3
C The femoral nerve roots originate from L1,2,3
D The femoral nerve supplies the whole quadriceps muscle group
E The hamstrings are supplied by the obturator nerve

Question 250

The cranial nerves

A The oculomotor nerve leaves the skull through the superior orbital fissure
B Trigeminal nerve injury will lead to loss of corneal reflexes
C Facial nerve injury can cause Bell's palsy
D Vagus nerve injury is associated with palate weakness
E Hypoglossal nerve injury is associated with tongue atrophy

Question 251

The following are associated with the temporal lobe

A Olfactory impulses
B Fear
C Gustatory impulses
D Visual impulses
E Memory recall

Question 252

A hypothalamic lesion will often cause the following

A Somnolence
B Disturbances of temperature regulation
C Disturbances of fat metabolism
D Dysmetria
E Disturbances in eating habits

Question 253

Structures passing through openings in the cranial floor are

A Ophthalmic artery—optic foramen
B Mandibular division—foramen ovale
C Vagus nerve—jugular foramen
D Internal carotid artery—foramen magnum
E Hypoglossal nerve—hypoglossal canal

Question 254

Drugs used as miotic agents to control intraocular pressure are

A Pilocarpine
B Atropine
C Phenylephrine
D Physostigmine
E Cocaine

Question 255

Absent knee jerks and extensor plantar reflexes in children are characteristic of

A Cord compression at L4/5
B Cerebral palsy
C Folate deficiency
D Friedreich's ataxia
E Vitamin B_{12} deficiency

Question 256

Are the following associations between cranial nerve nuclei and the origin of cranial nerves true or false?

A Medulla—eighth
B Midbrain—fourth
C Pons—seventh
D Corpus callosum—third
E Medulla—eleventh

Question 257

Ascending tracts and fibres of the spinal cord include the

A Posterior spinothalamic
B Spinoreticular
C Spino-olivary
D Corticospinal
E Spinotectal

Question 258

The basal ganglia include the following

A Substantia nigra
B Putamen
C Red nucleus
D Globus pallidus
E Caudate nucleus

Question 259

The grey matter is composed of the following

A Capillaries
B Fibre tracts
C Myelinated axons
D Nerve cells
E Unmyelinated axons

Question 260

True or false?

A Cortical release of GABA is increased during sleep
B Hypergabaergic activation in the pallidus can result in rigidity
C Release of GABA can be decreased by high extracellular potassium
D Glycine is involved in metabolism of peptides
E Glutamate has a powerful stimulatory effect

Question 261

Glutamate is characterised by

A Present only in cortical neurones
B Kainic acid as an agonist
C Decreased during viral encephalitis
D Increased release during sleep
E Release is calcium dependent

Question 262

Are the following associations between the structures and functions of neurones true or false?

A Cell membrane—excitation and transport
B Myelin—synaptic transmission
C Mitochondria—energy metabolism
D Lysosomes—secretion
E Nucleolus—Protein synthesis

Question 263

Are the following associations between reflexes and nerves true or false?

A Plantar—tibial
B Biceps—musculocutaneous
C Light—third cranial nerve
D Corneal—seventh cranial
E Triceps—median

Question 264

These are true about common neurotransmitters

A Acetylcholine is predominantly secreted by the neuromuscular junction
B Serotonin can be secreted by parasympathetic neurones
C Gamma-aminobutyric acid is found in cerebral cortex
D Dopamine can be secreted from hypothalamus
E Glycine can be found in the cerebral cortex

Question 265

True or false?

A The sciatic nerve arises from L3, 4, S1, 2
B The peroneal nerve supplies all the extensors of legs and feet
C Injuries to S1 may lead to lost sensation on the fifth toe
D The first lumbrical of the foot is supplied by the medial plantar nerve
E The seventh cranial nerve leaves the skull via the stylomastoid foramen

Neurology questions

Question 266

Duchenne muscular dystrophy

A May present as floppiness at birth
B Children who are delayed in walking by 18 months of age need to have CK measured
C EMG has no place in diagnosing DMD
D May be associated with IDDM
E The heart is often affected

Question 267

The following nerves contain preganglionic parasympathetic fibres as they leave the brain

A Oculomotor
B Trigeminal
C Facial
D Vagus
E Hypoglossal

Question 268

Down-beating nystagmus occurs with these conditions

A Niemann–Pick disease type C
B Cerebellar degeneration
C Demyelinating disorders
D Arnold–Chiari malformation
E Ataxia telangiectasia

Question 269

Nocturnal seizures are a manifestation of

A Landu–Kleffner syndrome
B Benign Rolandic epilepsy of childhood
C Hypopituitarism
D Glycogen storage disease type Ia
E Temporal lobe epilepsy syndrome

Question 270

Are the following statements about herpes encephalitis true or false?

A Can be caused by type 2 herpes virus
B EEG is abnormal even when cranial CT is normal
C May lead to epilepsy
D CSF will show lymphocytosis and low glucose
E 2 weeks of IV acyclovir and 2 weeks of oral acyclovir is the treatment of choice

Question 271

True or false?

A The muscles of the thenar eminence are supplied solely by the median nerve
B Paralysis of the lateral popliteal nerve causes loss of ankle jerks
C Injury to the radial nerve causes loss of first dorsal interosseus
D Sciatic nerve damage causes loss of dorsiflexion
E Femoral nerve damage causes adductor paralysis

Question 272

In dermatomyositis

A Distal weakness is one of the characteristic features
B There is an underlying malignancy in 30% of paediatric patients
C MRI is not helpful for diagnosis
D Prednisolone is the only treatment of choice
E Calcification occurs in two-thirds of children

Question 273

Juvenile myoclonic epilepsy

A Only occurs in boys
B Responds very well to carbamazepine
C Is not associated with generalised tonic/clonic seizures
D EEG is characterised by poly spike and waves
E Is a life-long problem

Question 274

True or false?

A The ulnar nerve originates from the lateral and medial cords
B Claw hand is a feature of median nerve injury
C The ulnar nerve supplies all the lumbricalis muscles
D The sensory distribution of the ulnar nerve is restricted to the dorsal and ventral areas of the little finger and the lateral aspect of the ring finger
E The median nerve supplies all the thenar muscles

Question 275

True or false?

A The hippocampus is the memory organ
B Frontal lobe lesions may present with violent behaviour
C Lesions in the hypothalamus are usually not associated with seizures
D Sleep EEG is of no value in myoclonic seizures
E Receptive dysphasia is associated with Landu–Kleffner syndrome

Question 276

The cortex of humans is characterised by

A Six bands or layers
B Neurones have only myelinated fibres
C Axon terminals are the main supply of neurotransmitters
D The dendritic structure of the newborn is mature
E The synapse is the structure through which signals are transmitted

Question 277

Lesions in white matter may be associated with the following conditions

A Acute demyelinating encephalomyelopathy
B Adrenal leukodystrophy
C Hemiplegia
D Gelastic seizures
E Huntington's chorea

Question 278

The characteristic features of tuberous sclerosis are

A Shagreen patches
B Angiomatosis
C Ash-leaf patches
D Axillary freckling
E Tramline appearance on skull X-ray

Question 279

Large pupils are commonly associated with

A Pontine haemorrhages
B Holmes–Adie syndrome
C Third nerve palsy
D Horner's syndrome
E Tricyclic antidepressant poisoning

Question 280

The GABA neurotransmitter

A Can be found in the peripheral nervous system
B Is degraded by transaminase
C Benzodiazepines increase affinity to GABA$_B$
D Beclofen is a selective GABA$_B$ agonist
E GABA$_B$ is mainly in the synaptic cleft

Question 281

N-Methyl-D-aspartate (NMDA) receptors are characterised by

A Action is blocked by magnesium
B Present in dorsal horn interneurones
C Involved in seizure activity
D Universal excitatory effects
E NMDA is a neurotransmitter

Question 282

Neurocutaneous disorders usually associated with seizures include

A Cavernous haemangioma
B Tuberous sclerosis
C Incontinentia pigmenti
D Sturge–Weber syndrome
E Albinism

Question 283

Are the following statements about sodium valproate true or false?

A Is not used for myoclonic seizures
B Has no effect on weight
C Cannot be given rectally
D Hypersensitivity is common
E Is associated with hirsutism

Question 284

Acute cerebellar ataxia is associated with the following conditions

A Astrocytoma
B Post chicken pox infection
C Migraine
D Seizures
E Carbamazepine toxicity

Question 285

Benign intracranial hypertension is associated with

A Sixth nerve palsy
B Papilloedema
C Early morning sickness
D Open pressure of 12 mmHg on lumbar puncture
E Treatment of newly diagnosed cystic fibrosis

Question 286

Are the following statements about Sydenham's chorea in children true or false?

A May follow streptococcal infection
B Movement can be more distally in limbs
C Speech is normal
D Involves the same muscle group
E Carbamazepine may be effective as treatment

Question 287

In acute transverse myelitis

A Lesions affect one side of the spinal cord
B There is often an association with viral infection
C Urinary retention is a prominent feature
D Sensory loss is almost always present
E High CSF protein is found in all cases

Question 288

The characteristic features on MRI of the following diseases are

A Optic neuritis—demyelination of optic tract
B Tuberous sclerosis—periventricular calcification
C Temporal lobe epilepsy—shrunken hippocampus
D Cerebral infarction—low signal on T2-weighted sequences
E Sturge–Weber syndrome—tramline appearance

Question 289

Absence epilepsy is characterised by

A Duration of absence of 1–2 minutes
B A postictal phase
C Hyperventilation usually precipitating typical absences
D Ictal EEG showing 3 Hz slow wave generalised activity without spikes
E Closed eyes during an attack

Question 290

Features of occipital lobe epilepsy of childhood may include

A Dominant visual symptoms
B Vomiting is not common
C Bilateral spike or slow waves on EEG when eyes are closed
D Good outcome
E Relationship to coeliac disease

Question 291

These are the main causes of neonatal seizures

A Hypoglycaemia
B Biotinidase deficiency
C Hyponatraemia
D Tuberous sclerosis
E Incontinentia pigmenti

Question 292

The following functional neuroimaging techniques may be used for presurgical assessment in epileptic patients

A Positron emission tomography (PET scan)
B Single photon emission computed tomography (SPECT)
C Magnetic resonance imaging (MRI)
D Magneto-encephalography (MEG)
E Computed tomography (CT)

Question 293

Are the following associations between anti-epileptic drugs and treatment or side effects true or false?

A Carbamazepine—myoclonic seizures
B Vigabatrin—visual field defect
C Ethosuximide—absence seizures
D Lamotrigine—partial seizures
E Topiramate—secondary generalised seizures

Question 294

True or false?

A Sudden death in epileptic patients may be due to apnoea
B The risk of relapse in the first year after stopping AED is about 60%
C The educational level of epileptic patients is lower than that of normal population
D Anti-epileptic drugs can be stopped after a seizure-free period of one year
E Contraceptive pills do not interfere with epilepsy treatment

Question 295

The following drugs can be used as prophylactic anti-migraine treatment

A Propanolol
B Phenytoin
C Clonidine
D Sumatriptan
E Nifedipine

Question 296

Occlusion of the cerebral arteries can cause infarction of the following areas

A Middle cerebral artery—internal capsule
B Posterior cerebral artery—occipital lobe
C Inferior cerebral artery—auditory cortex
D Meningeal artery—retinal haemorrhage
E Basilar artery—cord infarction

Question 297

Proximal muscle weakness occurs in

A Thyrotoxicosis
B Hypothyroidism
C Cushing's disease
D Conn's syndrome
E Familial hypokalaemic periodic paralysis

Question 298

Drugs which may precipitate myasthenia gravis include

A Succinyl choline
B Kanamycin
C Atropine
D Streptomycin
E Pyridostigmine

Infectious diseases questions

Question 299

Are the following associations between viruses and the diseases they cause true or false?

A Paramyxoviruses—respiratory syncytial disease
B Herpes virus—chorioretinitis
C Togaviruses—poliomyelitis
D Retroviruses—hepatitis A
E Rotavirus—infantile diarrhoea

Question 300

Are the following associations between types of rash and viral infections true or false?

A Maculopapular—rubella
B Petechial—chicken pox
C Vesicular—echovirus
D Telangiectatic—Coxsackie virus
E Urticarial—CMV

Question 301

Gram-positive bacteria include

A *Proteus vulgaris*
B *Listeria monocytogenes*
C Group B streptococci
D *Salmonella typhi*
E *Brucella canis*

Question 302

Are the following statements about beta-haemolytic streptococci true or false?

A The cell wall of group A has a polysaccharide layer
B The M protein layer has 20 different antigenic proteins
C Infection with one type of group A protects against infection by other streptococci
D The extracellular toxins they produce are responsible for fever
E Two streptolysins are produced by group A Beta haemolytic streptococci

Question 303

The bacteria that most commonly cause meningitis in the newborn are

A Meningococcus
B *E. coli*
C *Listeria monocytogenes*
D Group B streptococcus
E *Staphylococcus aureus*

Question 304

Common causes of bacterial meningitis at 4 years of age include

A *E. coli*
B Neisseria Meningitidis
C Streptoccus Pneumonia
D *Haemophilus influenzae*
E *Staphylococcus epidermidis*

Question 305

Are the following statements about *Corynebacterium diphtheriae* true or false?

A It is a Gram-negative club-shaped bacillus
B It usually produces a powerful exotoxin
C Of the three strains, the strongest is mitis
D Therapeutic agents can modify the fixation of toxin in tissue
E The membrane can extend up to the trachea

Question 306

Are the following statements about *Clostridium tetani* true or false?

A It is an anaerobic Gram-positive bacillus
B In wounds it produces enterotoxins
C It produces a toxin which abolishes the synaptic inhibition between neural end plate and anterior horn cells
D In tetanus, patients present with convulsions as the first symptom
E Human tetanus immune globulin is given IV in infection

Question 307

Bacterial infections which cause neutropenia include

A *Salmonella typhi* and *paratyphi*
B Shigellosis
C *Yersinia pestis*
D Brucellosis
E Leptospirosis

Question 308

Are the following statements about whooping cough true or false?

A *Bordetella pertussis* is a Gram-positive coccobacillus
B It is age specific
C It has three phases and they are 3 weeks apart
D Death is more common in the convalescent stage
E Erythromycin may eradicate the infection and halt its progression to other stages

Question 309

Complications related to infection with Meningococcus sepsis are

A Renal failure
B SIADH
C Arthritis
D Waterhouse–Friderichsen syndrome
E Subdural effusion

Question 310

The tuberculin skin test (Mantoux)

A Is done by injecting 0.1 ml of standard PPD subcutaneously
B Is a type III immune reaction
C Is negative in malnutrition
D The dilution commonly used is 1:1000
E An area of induration of at least 5 mm with erythema after 72 hours is positive

Question 311

Criteria in favour of diagnosing lepromatous leprosy include

A The centre of the macular lesion is anaesthetic
B Thickening of skin with many bacilli
C Low resistance to disease
D Vigorous cell-mediated immune response
E Leonine facies characteristic of advanced disease

Question 312

The following are criteria of legionnaires' disease

A It is caused by Gram-positive *L. pneumophila*
B Diarrhoea
C Proteinuria
D Neutropenia
E Mental confusion

Question 313

Common complications associated with measles infection include

A Giant-cell pneumonia in a leukaemic child
B Sensorineural deafness
C Cancrum oris
D Subacute sclerosing panencephalitis within 2 years
E Myocarditis

Question 314

True or false?

A 'Koplik's spots' are pathognomonic of measles
B By 12 years of age 50% of children demonstrate rubella antibodies
C Axillary lymph gland enlargement is seen before the rash in rubella infection
D Polyarthritis is a common sequel of rubella
E Immunity following herpes zoster infection is lifelong

Question 315

The following are characteristic features of herpes zoster (shingles)

A A non-immune child may develop shingles when exposed to chicken pox
B The virus remains in the sensory root ganglia of cord and brain
C Macules appear as the first sign
D It responds to acyclovir
E It is associated with post-herpetic neurological symptoms

Question 316

In respiratory syncytial virus infection (RSV)

A Haemagglutination can be produced
B Bronchiolitis is specifically caused by RSV
C Children below one year of age are usually affected
D There can be herpangina
E Keratoconjunctivitis is common

Question 317

The rash associated with typhoid fever

A Blanches on pressure
B Does not itch
C First appears on limbs
D Usually lasts one week
E Appears in the second week

Question 318

Clinical features associated with HBV and HAV infection are

A Conjugated jaundice
B Arthritis
C Constipation
D Urticarial rash
E Abdominal tenderness

Question 319

True or false?

A An infant whose mother is HBsAg positive during the third trimester should have HBIG after birth and 3 doses of vaccine
B Vaccinated persons should be tested for HBsAg and anti-HBs; if both are negative the test should be repeated after 4 weeks and the person should not be re-vaccinated
C The rate of success of active and passive immunisation in HBV is 60%
D Carriers of HBV can be treated with steroids
E There is no vaccine against HAV

Question 320

Complications that may follow paralytic poliomyelitis include

A Melaena
B Hypertension
C Hypercalciuria
D Myocarditis
E Gastric dilatation

Question 321

Are the following associations between antiviral drugs and viruses true or false?

A Amantadine—herpes simplex
B Acyclovir—varicella zoster
C Vidarabine—Coxsackie
D Ribavirin—RSV
E Ganciclovir—EPV

Question 322

Cat scratch disease

A Is caused by virus
B Can follow scratches by monkey
C There are painful papules in the early stages
D Axillary and inguinal lymph node enlargement is common
E Cefotaxime is effective

Question 323

Are the following associations between protozoan infections in children and characteristic features true or false?

A Amoebiasis—cysts or trophozoites on duodenal aspiration
B Giardiasis—transmitted by person to person contact
C Cryptosporodium—watery diarrhoea
D Plasmodium malaria—nephrotic syndrome
E Filariasis—mucusy diarrhoea

Question 324

Are the following associations between drugs and helminths true or false?

A Mebendazole—*E. vermicularis*
B Piperazine salts—strongyloidosis
C Ferrous sulphate—hook worms
D Diethylcarbamazine—*Toxocara canis*
E Praziquantel—paragonimiasis

Dermatology questions

Question 325

The following rashes are transient in a newborn baby

A Milia
B Cutis marmorata
C Subcutaneous fat necrosis
D Erythema toxicum neonatorum
E Port wine stain

Question 326

Are the following associations between nappy rashes and treatment in infants true or false?

A Seborrhoeic dermatitis—antibiotics
B Atopic eczema—hydrocortisone 1%
C Ammoniacal dermatitis—nystatin
D Candidiasis—amphotericin
E Napkin psoriasis—steroids

Question 327

The following features are characteristic of eczema in children

A It is associated with dermal oedema
B 70% of cases are familial
C In 50% of cases it will disappear by the age of 15 years
D It usually starts after the age of 3 months
E Environmental factors have no role in causing eczema

Question 328

Are the following associations between gastrointestinal diseases and skin abnormalities true or false?

A Coeliac disease—dermatitis herpetiformis
B Intestinal polyps in Peutz–Jeghers syndrome—telangiectasia
C Ulcerative colitis—fistula in ano
D Blind loop syndrome—scleroderma
E Crohn's disease—erythema nodosum

Question 329

Acneiform eruption may be associated with

A Tetracycline
B Prednisolone
C GH therapy
D Isoniazid
E Septrin

Question 330

Are the following associations between nail involvement and diseases true or false?

A Onycholysis—atopic eczema
B Nail pitting—trichinosis
C Splinter haemorrhage—subacute endocarditis
D Clubbing—cystic fibrosis
E Nail hypoplasia—Edwards' syndrome

Question 331

Are the following statements true of atopic eczema rather than seborrhoeic dermatitis?

A The child is irritable and itchy
B Mainly starts on the scalp and around genitalia
C Affects flexural and extensor areas
D May be associated with ichthyosis vulgaris
E Is associated with cradle cap

Question 332

Vulvovaginitis in schoolgirls may be due to

A Psychogenic causes
B Sexual abuse
C Haemorrhoids
D Thread worms
E Pediculosis

Question 333

Are the following associations between infectious organisms and skin diseases true or false?

A Human papillomavirus—molluscum contagiosum
B Pox virus—common warts
C Herpes virus—erythema multiforme
D *Staphylococcus epidermidis*—impetigo
E Paramyxovirus—whitlow

Question 334

The following are known causes of urticaria

A Codeine
B Urinary tract infection
C Strawberries
D Lymphomas
E Sunlight

Question 335

Are the following associations between skin diseases and infectious agents true or false?

A Pityriasis versicolor—*Trichophyton verrucosum*
B Erysipelas—*Staphylococcus aureus*
C Hand, foot and mouth disease—Coxsackie A16
D Folliculitis—streptococci
E Tinea capitis—*Malassezia furfur*

Question 336

Are the following associations between type of psoriasis and site true or false?

A Guttate—scalp
B Chronic plaque psoriasis—flexural sites
C Intertrigo—flexural sites
D Guttate—trunk
E Psoriatic arthropathy—terminal interphalanges

Question 337

Capillary haemangioma is associated with the following

A Kasabach–Merritt syndrome
B Sturge–Weber syndrome
C Salmon patch
D Klippel–Trenaunay–Weber syndrome
E Strawberry naevus

Question 338

The following changes in benign melanoma are used as evidence for diagnosing malignant melanoma

A Bleeding
B Variation in size and shape
C Infection
D Changes in colour
E Presence of hair

Question 339

Common causes of soft nodules are

A Exostosis
B Keloid
C Lipoma
D Neurofibroma
E Dermoid

Question 340

Hypermelanosis is usually associated with

A Biliary cirrhosis
B Eczema
C Pellagra
D Fanconi's syndrome
E Ultraviolet light therapy

Question 341

Are the following statements about human hair true or false?

A Daily hair loss is about 100 hairs
B Trichotillomania means falling out of hair due to radiotherapy
C Alopecia has increasing incidence of vitiligo
D Menke's "kinky hair" syndrome is an autosomal dominant disease
E Turner's syndrome is associated with hirsutism

Question 342

Are the following associations between syndromes and their inheritance true or false?

A Ichthyosis vulgaris—autosomal dominant
B Peutz–Jeghers syndrome—autosomal recessive
C Lamellar ichthyosis—X-linked recessive
D Fabry's disease—X-linked recessive
E Acrodermatitis enteropathica—autosomal recessive

Question 343

Skin diseases associated with the CNS are

A Sturge–Weber syndrome
B Neurofibromatosis type I
C Vitiligo
D Tuberous sclerosis
E McCune–Albright syndrome

Question 344

Are the following statements about normal skin true or false?

A Langerhans' cells play a role against infection
B Blood vessels, nerve fibres and sweat glands traverse the epidermis
C Collagen and reticulin are constituents of the subcutis layer
D Pilosebaceous glands are a constituent of the dermis
E Hair follicles lie in the subcutis layer

Joint and bone diseases questions

Question 345

In juvenile chronic arthritis (JCA)

A Rheumatoid factor is positive in systemic onset JCA
B A 15-year-old male with pauci-articular JCA will have positive rheumatoid factor
C ANA is positive in pauci-articular JCA in early childhood
D A child with positive rheumatoid factor has a poor prognosis
E HLA-B27 is associated with JCA

Question 346

The clinical presentation of rickets in infants and children is characterised by

A Bowing of the legs
B Widening of wrist bone
C Proximal myopathy
D Repeated fractures
E Tetany

Question 347

The commonest causes of chronic arthritis in childhood are

A Neuroblastoma
B Viral infection
C Mucocutaneous lymph node disease
D Hypogammaglobulinaemia
E Dermatomyositis

Question 348

In Perthé's disease

A Only obese girls are affected
B Disease is usually bilateral
C It is usually associated with painless limp
D Weight bearing is not allowed during the period of treatment
E Shortening of stature is very rare

Question 349

Are the following associations between parts of the cardiovascular system and collagen diseases affecting them true or false?

A Large arteries—Kawasaki disease
B Medium-sized arteries—PN
C Coronary artery aneurysm—Kawasaki disease
D Aortic arch arteritis—scleroderma
E Vasculitis—Henoch–Schönlein purpura

Question 350

Characteristic features of septic arthritis

A Joints are red, hot, swollen and painful
B The diagnostic test is joint aspiration
C High levels of glucose and white cells in synovial fluid
D Bone scan is invaluable
E May be caused by gonococcal infection

Question 351

Known causes of torticollis include

A Strabismus
B Klippel–Feil syndrome
C JCA
D Myositis
E Posterior fossa tumour

Question 352

Are the following statements about systemic onset JCA true or false?

A Enlargement of lymph nodes is common
B Pericarditis is not uncommon
C Joint involvement is symmetrical
D A normal ESR virtually excludes the diagnosis
E There is hypogammaglobulinaemia

Question 353

Are the following associations between drugs used in treatment of JCA and side effects true or false?

A Ibuprofen—gastritis
B Naproxen—neutropenia
C Aspirin—exacerbation of asthma
D Hydroxychloroquine—retinopathy
E Indomethacin—renal failure

Question 354

Are the following associations between these conditions and clinical presentations true or false?

A Polyarteritis nodosa—eosinophilia
B Takayasu arteritis—pulseless disease
C SLE—multiple organ infarction
D Scleroderma—morphoea
E Kawasaki disease—Raynaud's phenomenon

Question 355

Diagnostic criteria of Kawasaki disease are

A Conjunctivitis and cracking of the lips
B Cervical lymphadenopathy
C High fever for 5 days
D Leukocytosis
E Arthritis

Question 356

Common causes of scoliosis in children are

A Postural
B Duchenne muscular dystrophy
C Tuberculosis
D Neurofibromatosis
E Spina bifida

Question 357

Characteristic features of achondroplasia are

A 80% of cases are new mutations
B Increase in lumbar interpedicular distance on spinal X-ray
C Hands are short while trunk is normal in length
D Hydrocephalus is rare
E Defect in proliferation of cartilage and normal membranous bone formation

Question 358

Are the following associations between syndromes and bony defects true or false?

A Ellis–van Creveld—polydactyly
B Jeune's syndrome—narrow immobile chest
C Osteopetrosis—pancytopenia
D Pyknodysostosis—repeated fractures
E Caffey's disease—cortical thickening

Question 359

The following syndromes are commonly associated with syndactyly

A Laurence–Moon–Biedl
B Apert's
C Pfeiffer's
D Poland's
E Rubinstein–Taybi

Eyes, ears, nose and throat questions

Question 360

Corneal deposition is associated with the following disorders

A Hunter's syndrome
B Morquio's syndrome
C Rubella syndrome
D Cystinosis
E Hurler's syndrome

Question 361

Cataracts are commonly associated with

A Galactosaemia
B Amiodarone
C Down's syndrome
D Steroids
E Glaucoma

Question 362

Amblyopia

A Is usually bilateral
B Visual acuity is decreased
C Crowding phenomenon is common
D Results in progressive loss of vision
E May be caused by malnutrition

Question 363

Impairment of accommodation can be associated with

A Atropine poisoning
B Wilson's disease
C Diabetes mellitus
D Ptosis
E Botulism

Question 364

Total loss of vision (amaurosis) may be due to

A Anoxia
B Papilloedema
C Craniopharyngioma
D Chorioretinitis
E Retinal detachment

Question 365

Paralytic squint

A Deviation is worse on gaze into the field of action of the affected muscle
B Is associated with diplopia on looking away from the affected eye
C Is associated with torticollis
D Is the commonest type at all ages
E There is no fixation on cover test

Question 366

Are the following associations between syndromes affecting the eyes and clinical features true or false?

A Duane—retraction of the globe on abduction
B Mobius—abduction weakness
C Gradenigo—congenital abducens nerve palsy
D Parinaud—horizontal gaze palsy
E Brown—elevation of the eye on abduction is absent

Question 367

The commonest causes of ophthalmia neonatorum are

A A gonococcal infection caused by *Neisseria meningitidis* in the first 2–3 days
B Chlamydia in the first 24 hours
C Chemical after 7 days
D *Staphylococcus aureus* in the first 2–3 days
E Herpes simplex in the first week

Question 368

Ectopia lentis

A Is rare following trauma
B In Marfan's syndrome lens dislocation is outward and inward
C In homocystinuria lens dislocation is inward and outward
D Is associated with aniridia
E Is commonly caused by microcornea

Question 369

In optic atrophy

A Homonymous hemianopia is common
B A white optic disc is the characteristic feature
C It is usually associated with hydrocephalus
D Mitochondrial degenerative diseases are a common cause
E There is associated retraction of the globe

Question 370

Orbital cellulitis is caused by

A *Haemophilus influenzae* type b
B *Staphylococcus aureus*
C Group B beta-haemolytic streptococcus
D *Streptococcus pneumoniae*
E Actinomycosis

Question 371

Risk factors constituting an indication for neonatal screening for hearing loss include

A Family history
B Birth weight <1500 grams
C Congenital infection
D Neonatal jaundice associated with prematurity
E More than 10 days on mechanical ventilation during the neonatal period

Question 372

The ages at which infants and children respond well to hearing tests are

A 0–4 weeks—momentarily stop activity in response to sounds
B 5–6 months—localised sounds in the horizontal plane
C 2 years—speech audiometry
D 5 years—Stycar picture
E 7 years—pure-tone audiometry

Question 373

The following are recognised features of otitis externa

A Itching
B Hearing loss
C Bulging tympanic membrane
D Invariably associated with fever
E Topical antibiotics and steroids are effective

Question 374

Are the following statements about sinuses and sinusitis true or false?

A The frontal sinus is the first to develop in infants
B Peri-orbital oedema and facial pain are commonly associated with sinusitis
C Headache is a common feature of sinusitis
D Ethmoiditis is a common cause of peri-orbital cellulitis
E Sinus X-ray is diagnostic of sinusitis

Oncology questions

Question 375

Clinical manifestations of ALL which are usually found at first presentation include

A Bone and joint pain
B Lethargy and weakness
C Cervical lymph node enlargement
D Jaundice
E Dyspnoea

Question 376

Morphology of lymphoblasts in ALL

A More than 80% have a chromosomal abnormality
B Most cases have the phenotype of immature B cells
C Have a high cytoplasmic to nuclear ratio
D Are sudan black and peroxidase positive
E About 15% have a T cell phenotype

Question 377

Myeloblastic leukaemia

A Is more common in younger age groups
B Bleeding is a common presentation
C Lymphadenopathy is one of the characteristic features
D Long-term survival can be achieved in 40–50% of patients
E At least 10% of leukaemic blast cells should be present in the bone marrow

Question 378

The FAB (French American British) classification of AML

A Is associated with 7 types of cells
B M1 has blast cells that are sudan black/peroxidase negative
C M3 is characterised by promyelocytic cells and bleeding gums
D M5 has monocytic type cells
E In M6 about 30% of marrow cells are erythroblasts with few myeloblasts

Question 379

Hodgkin's lymphoma

A Is more common in boys
B Reed–Sternberg cells in bone marrow are pathognomonic
C Most commonly presents with generalised lymphadenopathy
D Anaemia can present early
E The lymphocyte predominant type has a good prognosis

Question 380

Poor prognostic features in Hodgkin's lymphoma are

A High ESR
B Absence of systemic symptoms
C Low lymphocyte count
D Mediastinal mass
E Anaemia

Question 381

Are the following statements about Hodgkin's lymphoma true or false?

A Stage II: two or more nodes affected on both sides of the abdomen
B Stage IB: a single lymph node region without temperature or weight loss
C Radiotherapy is given to all patients with HD
D The second commonest malignant tumour associated with HD is AML
E Complete remission is achieved in 90% of patients with modern treatment

Question 382

Non-Hodgkin lymphoma

A Is mostly a T-cell lymphoma
B Generalised lymphadenopathy with hepatosplenomegaly is common
C Autoimmune haemolytic anaemia is common
D In the low-grade type, small and follicular cells are predominant
E 2-year survival is achieved in 90% of patients with therapy

Question 383

In insulinoma

A Low blood glucose with high insulin level is pathognomonic
B The pro-insulin level is elevated
C May be familial (Werner's syndrome)
D Symptoms can be controlled by diazoxide
E Total pancreatectomy with insulin replacement is the treatment of choice

Question 384

Are the following statements about malignancy in children true or false?

A There is an increased incidence of leukaemia after exposure to atomic radiation
B Radiotherapy for non-malignant conditions carries no risk
C Diethylstilbestrol is carcinogenic
D Immunosuppressive therapy does not increase risk of malignancy in children
E Intrauterine exposure to X-rays of 3 rads may cause tumour

Question 385

Are the following statements about treatment of ALL true or false?

A IV administration of chemotherapy drugs can achieve therapeutic CNS concentrations
B Cranial irradiation has no long-term effects
C Intrathecal chemotherapy may cause meningitis
D Cranial nerve palsy is very commonly due to chemotherapy
E Relapse in liver and lymph nodes is not very common

Question 386

Are the following statements about histiocytosis true or false?

A There is skin involvement in 50% of cases of Langerhans' cell histiocytosis
B Skin lesions are haemorrhagic
C Diabetes insipidus is always present in LCH
D 65% of children under 2 years of age with no organ dysfunction survive for 5 years
E Single agent chemotherapy is effective in LCH

Question 387

The following are used in treatment of neuroblastoma

A Surgery
B Chemotherapy is not effective in rapidly disseminated tumour
C Most neuroblastomas are not radiosensitive
D MIBG (metaiodobenzylguanidine) is used in treatment
E Mass screening of 6-month-old babies by urine VMA is not useful in early detection of neuroblastoma

Question 388

Wilms' tumour is associated with

A Genitourinary anomalies
B Aniridia
C A deletion on chromosome 13q
D Hemihypertrophy
E Neuroblastoma

Question 389

Recognised features of rhabdomyosarcoma are

A Painless mass
B Epistaxis
C Cranial nerve palsy
D Hypercalcaemia
E Vaginal bleeding

Question 390

True or false?

A The standard treatment for unilateral retinoblastoma is enucleation
B Chemotherapy not effective for retinoblastoma localised to the globe
C The overall survival rate in retinoblastoma is 90%
D 80% of the inherited type retinoblastoma is bilateral at time of diagnosis
E Alpha fetoprotein is normal in retinoblastoma

Community paediatrics questions

Question 391

In infancy, findings strongly connected with abuse are

A Tear of frenulum of upper lip
B Parietal bone skull fracture
C Retinal haemorrhage
D Greenstick fracture of radius or ulna
E Burns on the back of the hand

Question 392

The following are good clinical markers of sexual abuse

A UTI in girls
B Encopresis in boys
C Laceration of penis
D Anogenital warts
E Daytime wetting

Question 393

Which of the following general statements about CSA are true?

A Most abuse is perpetrated by casual acquaintances
B Women rarely abuse children
C 15–20% of physically abused children are also sexually abused.
D 50% of deaf children are abused
E In 25% of cases the child's disclosure is false

Question 394

Criteria used to define screening procedures

A The incidence of the disease should be 1 in 2000 of the population
B The condition must be treatable
C The test is acceptable to the whole population
D The natural history of the condition is not important
E The test must be diagnostic of the condition

Question 395

Child protection conferences

A Are almost always held when a child has been abused
B Reports should be made available to all parties in care proceedings
C A doctor's presence is not usually required
D Parents should not be invited
E Decides when a child should be removed from his family

Question 396

True or false?

A Yellow colour of a bruise indicates that it is 13–15 days old
B Write down your opinion when you see an abused child
C Take the child's hospital notes with you when you give evidence in court
D Sexually abused children can be examined only if a parent is present
E Informed consent is required for each examination you perform on any child

Question 397

The chi-square test is

A Applied to a percentage
B Applied only to absolute numbers
C Never applied to proportion
D Equal to χ^2
E More sensitive than a student test

Question 398

Standard deviation (SD)

A Is the square root of variance
B 1 SD + or – mean = 95% of values fall within that range
C Is the basis of the chi-square test
D Is more than the standard error of the mean
E Is only of value for samples of small numbers

Question 399

Are the following statements about enuresis true or false?

A It can be caused by infection
B If it follows normal micturition it is psychogenic
C Urography and cystoscopy are usually performed as the first line of investigation
D Neurotic children have poor school performance
E Waking the child repeatedly at night is a means of treatment

Question 400

Are the following statements about encopresis true or false?

A It is more common in males
B It is the passage of faeces in inappropriate places
C Social problems are more commonly associated with encopresis than with enuresis
D Overflow incontinence indicates an organic defect
E Laxatives can be useful in its treatment

Question 401

Drugs that should be avoided during breast-feeding are

A Cimetidine
B Metronidazole
C Digoxin
D Tetracycline
E Bromocriptine

Question 402

Drugs that are safe during breast-feeding include

A Anaesthetic drugs
B Aldomet
C Phenobarbitone
D Propranolol
E Chloramphenicol

Question 403

Feeding problems in infancy can be due to

A Metabolic disorders
B Cystic fibrosis
C Constipation
D Tracheo-oesophageal fistula
E Maternal anxiety

Answers

Neonatology answers

Answer 1
A False   Can be used in late deceleration.
B True
C False   Abnormal foetal heart rate (bradycardia or tachycardia).
D False   Following acceleration of foetal heart rate.
E True

Answer 2
A True
B True   And also from mesoderm.
C False   From mesoderm.
D False   From mesoderm.
E True

Answer 3
A False   From conception to 8 weeks.
B True
C True
D False   The foetus grows at a rate of 1.5 mm/day.
E False   The embryonic heart starts beating at 7–8 weeks after
             conception.

Answer 4
A True   May be caused by pressure in birth canal, cord around neck.
            There are no long-term complications and no treatment is
            required.
B True   This may lead to unconjugated hyperbilirubinaemia and drop in
            haemoglobin.
C True   This usually disappears in the first two weeks of life and there
            are no long-term complications.
D False   No surgical decompression is needed. Care of the eyes is
             required. If abnormalities do not resolve, the mouth is deviated
             to one side and there is difficulty in closing the affected eye,
             then referral to a plastic surgeon is required.
E False   The lesion is at C8 and T1.

Answer 5

A True

B False   They have a poor sucking reflex and are floppy.

C True

D False   Tone is increased in legs rather than arms, which become normal in tone within the first weeks of life. A few newborn babies with moderate HIE may develop spastic diplegia or quadriplegia or hemiplegia.

E False   Only with severe form of HIE.

Answer 6

A False

B True   Much better than phenytoin.

C True   Has been used in older children with refractory status epilepticus and has proved to be effective in some cases.

D True   It can be used but should be accompanied by continuous EEG monitoring. The muscle twitches can always be controlled by IV phenobarbital, clonazepam or vecuronium but there are always subtle seizures and continuing brain activity. The best thing is to try to avoid paralysing agents such as vecuronium and use anticonvulsants in even higher doses in a controlled situation. EEG monitoring is recommended.

E False   There are benzodiazepine receptors in the brain.

Answer 7

A False   It also occurs with congenital pneumonia and meconium aspiration.

B True

C False   This may indicate infection, intraventricular haemorrhage, patent ductus arteriosus or a mechanical ventilatory problem.

D False   This is usually given to mothers; it is of no benefit if given to babies.

E False   Only a third of premature babies may need more than two doses of surfactant.

Answer 8

A True

B True   Can be used for babies of any size. In Scandinavian countries CPAP is used as the first line of ventilation in all premature babies.

C False   In acute collapse CPAP is not useful; it is best to use IPPV.

D True

E True   This is the commonest weaning process used in neonatal units in the UK.

Answer 9

A True   It has also been used as a rescue treatment in the management of pulmonary haemorrhage.

B False   It reduces the incidence of PBD.

C True

D True

E False   If given in a controlled aseptic way it will not increase the incidence of infection.

Answer 10

A False   It can occur in association with many conditions, e.g. lung immaturity or chronic diseases, hydrocephalus and intraventricular haemorrhage, gastro-oesophageal reflux and sepsis.

B False   It is usually cessation of breathing for 20–30 s with bradycardia and central cyanosis.

C True

D True   Obstructive apnoea is due to cessation of airflow.

E False   The association is not strong, but there is an association between central apnoea and SIDS.

Answer 11

A False   Hypoglycaemia occurs more often in babies that are small for gestational age and in large babies.

B False   Can happen in both.

C False   Associated with both.

D False   More common in small for gestational age infants and those with a diabetic mother.

E False   More common in premature babies.

Answer 12

A True   May lead to renal failure.

B True   Prevents platelet aggregation.

C False   Less than 7 days.

D True   May worsen the bleeding.

E False   Used if urine output is 1.6 ml/kg/hr.

Answer 13

A False   It is right ventricular hypertrophy.

B True

C True

D False   It is associated with right bundle branch block.

E False   Normal for age.

Answer 14
A False Unconjugated.
B True The most important condition to exclude is biliary atresia. There is a greater chance of a normal life and healthy liver if portoenterostomy (Kasai operation) is carried out before the age of 70 days. Other conditions include congenital infections, agenesis of gall bladder.
C False Unconjugated.
D True
E False Unconjugated.

Answer 15
A True Maternal SLE and sepsis may also cause thrombocytopenia.
B True Massive cutaneous haemangioma consumes the platelets.
C True When given to pregnant mother to control pregnancy induced hypertension.
D False This is a problem of platelet function, not count.
E True The baby will have maternal platelet antibodies.

Answer 16
A True It usually follows grade II–IV intraventricular haemorrhage.
B True It may cause vasoconstriction due to loss of blood.
C True It is very rare and not extensive.
D False It is usually germinal.
E False It depends on the size, site and association with other problems such as hydrocephalus.

Answer 17
A True Due to thrombosis.
B True Due to ischaemia.
C False Not common.
D True Due to ischaemia.
E True Multifactorial such as ischaemia, thrombosis, and toxins.

Answer 18
A False Uncommon with rubella; very common with CMV.
B True
C False This is an early manifestation; most of the time it is diagnosed at birth. The damage is permanent.
D False May be a late manifestation but is uncommon.
E False Presents earlier. The damage is permanent.

Answer 19
A True
B False Presents mainly with renal failure and loin mass.
C False Always presents with heavy proteinuria and sometimes with hydrops foetalis.
D True May occur secondary to severe sepsis or increased platelet consumption.
E False CMV can cause interstitial nephritis but haematuria is an uncommon presentation.

Answer 20
A True
B True Oxygen toxicity is the main cause of retinopathy of prematurity.
C False Low pH (acidosis).
D True The reason for this is not clear.
E False High PCO_2 may cause vasoconstriction of retinal blood vessels.

Answer 21
A True
B False IgM never crosses the placenta. If found in a newborn baby it is an indication that the newborn is suffering from a congenital infection.
C False All IgG subclasses are low.
D True
E True

Answer 22
A True
B True Newborn babies whose mother is infected within a week before and after delivery should be given herpes zoster immunoglobulin plus vaccination.
C False Persistently positive IgM in a baby indicates congenital infection. Transient positive IgM indicates that the mother has been infected with toxoplasmosis; no prenatal timing of infection can be given.
D False It is not a conclusive test. Diagnosis depends on the clinical picture with virus isolation and determination of T-cell subsets as the CD4:CD8 ratio is reversed.
E True

Answer 23

A True The range for diagnosing hypoglycaemia is between 2.1 and 2.6 mmol/l.

B True

C False

D False The standard dose is 2 ml/kg of 10% dextrose or infusion of glucose at a rate of 8 mmol/kg/h.

E False The number of insulin receptors is higher and that is why the newborn baby of a diabetic mother will suffer from resistant hypoglycaemia.

Answer 24

A True Especially if given just before delivery to a pregnant woman with pregnancy induced hypertension.

B False

C True

D False Not known.

E False May cause hyperglycaemia.

Answer 25

A True As well as hypercalcaemia.

B False Associated with babies on formula milk.

C False Associated with hypophosphaturia.

D False Associated with babies who are on formula milk.

E True

Genetics answers

Answer 26

A False The chromosomes are in the nucleus.
B True
C False This is translocation. A mutation is caused by loss of DNA arrangement of a single base pair.
D False A mutation causes considerable disturbance of cell function.
E False

Answer 27

A True
B False Xq21.
C True
D False 11.
E True Long arm of chromosome 13.

Answer 28

A False Autosomal recessive.
B False Autosomal recessive.
C True
D True
E True

Answer 29

A False Occurs in 25% of siblings if both parents are carriers.
B True Parents are carriers and rarely manifest the disease.
C False Occurs equally in females and males.
D True
E True

Answer 30

A False Associated with cataract, squint.
B False Not usually associated with fractures, but atlanto-axial dislocation is common.
C True
D False Males are infertile while females may be normal in translocation or mosaic.
E True

Answer 31

A False   Occurs in both.
B True
C False   Occurs in both.
D False   Is associated with trisomy 18.
E True

Answer 32

A True
B True   Associated with cleft lip and palate.
C False   Not reported.
D False   Warfarin is associated with high perinatal mortality and anomalies.
E True   May be associated with retarded skeletal growth, coloured teeth, cataract, and limb malformations.

Answer 33

A True   Foetal alcohol syndrome is characterised by dysmorphic features including long philtrum, smooth upper lip and microcephaly. Other features include coarctation of aorta, growth retardation and learning difficulties.
B False   Cigarette smoking is associated with intrauterine growth retardation and sudden infant death syndrome.
C True   Sacral agenesis.
D True   Developmental delay and seizures are other features.
E False   May be associated with small for gestation babies. Cocaine and heroin are associated with bleeding problems, which may lead to the baby being born with a cerebral infarct.

Answer 34

A False   Associated with microcephaly and periventricular calcification on cranial ultrasound or cranial computed tomography.
B True
C False   May be associated with systemic manifestations such as encephalitis.
D True   As hydrops foetalis.
E False   Deafness is commonly associated with rubella infection.

Answer 35
A True As well as refractory epilepsy.
B True Progressive motor neurone degeneration is associated with severe arthrogryposis and congenital anomalies of many organs.
C False
D False
E False Characterised by short stature, frontal bossing, small triangular facies, sparse subcutaneous tissue and, in many cases, hemihypertrophy.

Answer 36
A False Hurler's syndrome is a mucopolysaccharidosis with skeletal abnormalities, coarse facial features, cataract and short stature.
B False
C True Also associated with exomphalos, creases on ears and neonatal hypoglycaemia.
D False There are coarse facial features but not macroglossia.
E True Usually due to small oral cavity.

Answer 37
A True Also associated with polydactyly and retinitis pigmentosa.
B False Features of Goldenhaar syndrome are coloboma of iris and retina and deafness.
C False Ageing features.
D True
E True Also associated with diamond shaped eyes and small feet.

Answer 38
A False
B False Associated with trisomy 13.
C True
D True
E True

Answer 39
A True And 10% after second affected child. Prophylactic folic acid given to a high-risk mother reduces the risk of spina bifida to <2%.
B False
C True
D False The reconstruction of meningocele can be done early and children may live longer with other complications such as bladder and bowel problems and hydrocephalus.
E True Spinal dysraphism may present late or early with unilateral weakness and toileting problems.

Answer 40

A True   Also Laurence–Moon–Biedl syndrome.
B False   Associated with glaucoma and cataract.
C False   Mainly cataract but not common.
D False   May be associated with optic nerve glioma.
E True

Answer 41

A False   Usually pulmonary artery stenosis, VSD and cardiomyopathy.
B False
C True   Females are fertile, males infertile (cryptorchidism).
D True
E False   It is inherited as autosomal dominant with normal cognitive development.

Answer 42

A True   Has a bearing on parental understanding of child's needs and suitable environment.

B False   Has no effect on child development in a suitable environment.

C False

D True   Malnourished children can catch up very quickly with their peers if nutritional status is improved.

E True   e.g. cocaine, heroin.

Answer 43

A False   Adopted children do very well if a suitable environment is found.

B False   Neither large nor small families affect child development.

C True

D True   Very difficult to prove except by changing the environment.

E True   The main factor in most socially deprived families.

Answer 44

A True   Most infants will have good head control by the age of 3 months.

B True   Children with spastic cerebral palsy may do the same.

C False   Children only follow objects and fixate at this distance at the age of 6 months.

D False   This will start at around the age of 5–6 months.

E True   This may be the way to test hearing.

Answer 45

A True   Finger grasp (index and thumb) achieved at age of 10 months.

B False

C True   May stand and walk with support, depending upon ethnic origin.

D True   Also babbling noises "dada", "mama".

E True

Answer 46

A False   Walks up stairs using four limbs but needs help to come down stairs.

B True   Up to 30 single recognisable words in some children but majority can say between 3 and 10 single recognisable words.

C True   Circle by 2 years, cross by 3 years, square by 3½ years and triangle by 4–4½ years.

D True

E False   Achieved by the age of 2½ years.

Answer 47

A True   Can also recognise colours, her/his full name.
B False This will be achieved by age of 3 years, hops by 4 years.
C True
D True   Is also dry by day; still a few wet nappies at night.
E False May happen at the age of 4 years.

Answer 48

A False
B True   They do not crawl and are late in walking.
C True   2–5% at age 7–15 years.
D False This occurs earlier at the age of 2½ years.
E True   They can ride a tricycle by the age of 2½–3 years.

Answer 49

A False Very rare. The commonest cause of delayed speech is familial.
B True
C False Has no implication for speech and surgery is rarely required.
D True   Hearing must be checked in all children with delayed speech.
E True

Answer 50

A True   Other reasons include bullying at school or home, visual problems, dyspraxia for letters.
B False
C True
D True
E True   As with writing.

Answer 51

A False The mechanism is negative feedback.
B True
C False Secretion takes place in the form of pulses; continuous secretion inhibits gonadotrophins.
D True
E False LH is secreted at night in early puberty but during the daytime in late puberty.

Answer 52

A True
B False This is stage 2. In stage 3 the hair is dark and coarse.
C False This is stage 5 breast development. Stage 4 is characterised by projection of areola and papilla.
D True
E True

Answer 53

A False Occurs in both males and females.
B False Occurs in both males and females.
C False Very rarely causes precocious puberty in either sex.
D False
E True

Answer 54

A False Defined as height below the 3rd centile of age.
B True
C False It is consistent with chronological age.
D False Velocity over 1 year predicts the final height.
E True

Answer 55

A True
B True
C True
D True
E False Children with hypopituitarism will be normal in height at birth but 50% will present in the first year of life as not achieving the normal height for this age group.

Emergencies and resuscitation answers

Answer 56

A True No longer in the asystole protocol but can be considered as an additional drug where there is evidence of increased vagal tone as in intubation.

B False Always treat the cause; the commonest cause is usually hypoxia.

C False Dose is 20 mcg/kg; minimum total dose of 1 mcg can be used in children, and maximum is 2 mcg/dose in adolescents.

D False

E True Especially during elective intubation in neonates and children.

Answer 57

A True Due to various causes including diarrhoea, bleeding, burns, peritonitis, vomiting and sepsis.

B False Not common, but may cause hypovolaemic shock.

C True Trauma is one of the commonest causes of shock and may cause tension pneumothorax and haemopneumothorax.

D False Can cause cardiogenic shock but not common.

E False

Answer 58

A False Colloids more effectively expand intravascular volume.

B False Crystalloid first, followed by blood if needed.

C False Dextrose/saline solution can be given but not as a resuscitating fluid.

D True 10 ml/kg for neonates.

E True

Answer 59

A True The adrenergic effects are increased heart rate, myocardial contractility, and increased peripheral vascular resistance.

B False May cause peripheral vasoconstriction and arrhythmias.

C True Adrenaline is indicated as an infusion when other inotropes have failed in young infants and children with chronic heart disease.

D False

E True

Answer 60

A False   It increases myocardial contractility.
B True   A beta sympathomimetic reaction.
C False
D False   Sodium bicarbonate inactivates adrenaline and dopamine, and therefore the line must be flushed with saline if these drugs are subsequently given.
E True   Correcting acidosis will enhance the efficiency of adrenaline.

Answer 61

A False   It is recommended if there is no venous or intraosseous route within the first minute of resuscitation.
B True   Or 10 mcg/kg of 1:1000 in children.
C True
D True   You can give ten times of the first IV dose (100 mcg/kg of 1:10.000).
E False   Can be given. If adrenaline is required to sustain myocardial contractility, the outlook is usually poor.

Answer 62

A True
B True   This may lead to respiratory acidosis.
C True   To help clearance of CO_2.
D True   If it is respiratory acidosis.
E False   Low blood pressure makes acidosis worse.

Answer 63

A False
B True   1 mmol/kg/dose of 4.2% in children and 1–2 mmol/kg/dose in neonates.
C False   It can be given in an emergency. The UVC should be 3–4 cm from the umbilicus.
D True   The line should be infused with saline if adrenaline will be given after bicarbonate has been given.
E True   Especially in neonatal resuscitation.

Answer 64

A False   To the right.
B False   It is used in treatment of hyperkalaemia. After correction of acidosis, the potassium level falls because of intracellular movement and supplementation is required.
C True   In exchange for calcium it may cause hypocalcaemia.
D True
E True   There is a lot of NaCl in 8.4% of $NaHCO_3$.

Answer 65

A False
B True   Prostaglandin can be used to keep the duct open in aortic atresia, hypoplastic left heart syndrome, coarctation of aorta, transposition of the great arteries and tricuspid atresia. The side effect is apnoea, which should be controlled by ventilation if needed.
C True
D False
E True

Answer 66

A True   In high doses it may cause renal artery constriction.
B False   In low dose it is ineffective in children with chronic heart diseases.
C False   Causes vasoconstriction; this increases the blood pressure.
D True   Indirectly through cardiac beta adrenergic receptors.
E False

Answer 67

A True   It does not depend on endogenous noradrenaline and has direct action on catecholamine.
B False   Probably reduces the splanchnic blood flow.
C True   By increasing myocardial contractility and heart rate.
D False
E False   It has little effect on peripheral vascular tone.

Answer 68

A True   It can be given via ETT if there is no venous access.
B True
C True   It can also be used via a nebuliser in chronic asthma.
D False
E False

Answer 69

A True   The sino-atrial node is situated in the right atrium.
B False   The AV node further spreads depolarisation through specialised conducting tissue (His–Purkinje system).
C False   The AV node and bundle of His are situated in the lower part of the right atrium. Depolarisation spreads distally from the AV junction through two specialised bundles of conducting tissue (right and left), which in turn divide into a network of Purkinje fibres that supply the right and left ventricle.
D True   Depolarisation of the atria is recorded on the ECG as a deflection.
E True

Answer 70

A True
B True
C True   Also occur in systemic illness or following cardiac surgery involving the atria. Acute causes include abdominal distension, increased intracranial pressure, seizures, suctioning, endotracheal intubation and drugs such as digoxin, beta blockers, and verapamil.
D True
E True

Answer 71

A True
B False   May cause cardiac arrrest but is not common.
C True   The main cause of cardiac arrest in children is hypoxia and causes of hypoxia.
D True   May cause hypoxia.
E False

Answer 72

A True
B False   It will help to maintain tidal volume (8 ml/kg).
C True
D False   It can be used at any age but is sometimes difficult to use in children under 1 year of age as it is difficult to lift the epiglottis.
E True

Immunology and allergy answers

Answer 73

A True Antibodies accelerate the rate of activation of alternative pathway. The pathway may also be activated in the absence of antibodies. Both the alternative and classical pathways can activate C3.

B False The two main functions of T-cells are: (1) to signal B-cells to make antibody by producing cytokines and membrane molecules that can serve as ligands for B-cell surface molecules; (2) to kill virally infected cells or tumour cells.

C True

D True

E False IFNα and β inhibit viral replication, inhibit cell proliferation, activate natural killer cells and upregulate class I MHC.

Answer 74

A True

B False The principal phagocytes are neutrophils and monocytes in acute inflammation and microbial killing, and monocytes in chronic inflammation. Eosinophils are involved in allergic and parasitic responses.

C False The alternative pathway uses C3bBD–C356789 and the classical pathway uses C142356789.

D True

E False Cellular immunity.

Answer 75

A False X-linked recessive. It is characterised by atopic eczema, dermatitis, thrombocytopenic purpura with small defective platelets and susceptibility to infection. The gene is on the proximal arm of the X chromosome at Xp11.22–11.23.

B True

C False The T-cell reaction is reduced with monoclonal antibodies to CD3, CD4, and CD8.

D True Low serum IgM and high serum IgE. Normal or low IgG concentration, IgG subclasses normal.

E False

Answer 76

A True Infection may be caused by pneumococci, streptococci and *Haemophilus influenzae* but not by viruses or fungi.

B True Hypoplasia of adenoids, tonsils and peripheral lymph nodes is the rule in this condition.

C True

D True

E False Is usually given every 3–4 weeks.

Answer 77

A False X-linked recessive. The gene on the X chromosome is proximal to the muscular dystrophy gene and distal to ornithine transcarbamylase on Xp21.

B True Hydrogen peroxide and hydroxyl radicals that kill catalase-positive organisms are not produced in CGD.

C True

D True

E False There is a reservoir of cytochrome b, up to 80–90% found in neutrophil-specific granules.

Answer 78

A True Or umbilical cord infection in the neonatal period.

B False Associated with soft tissue infection such as otitis media, pharyngitis, stomatitis, cellulitis, perirectal abscess and recurrent bronchopneumonia as well as aseptic meningitis.

C False It is due to the absence or diminished expression of adhesive glycoproteins or carbohydrate ligands on the leukocyte surface.

D True There is defective expression of three α-β heterodimeric glycoprotein molecules unique to leukocytes.

E False

Answer 79

A True

B True

C True B-cells are high in X-linked SCID and T-cells are low in all types of SCID.

D False All SCID types are correctable by bone marrow transplantation.

E True There is absence of T- and B-cell function from birth.

Answer 80

A True   It is the prominent feature together with oculocutaneous telangiectasia, chronic sinopulmonary disease, a high incidence of malignancy and variable humoral and cellular immunodeficiency.

B True

C False   The abnormal gene has been mapped to the long arm of chromosome 11(11q22–23). There is increase in sensitivity to ionising radiation, defective DNA repair and frequent chromosomal abnormalities.

D True

E False

Answer 81

A True   Neutrophils of patients with CGD demonstrate normal chemotaxis, phagocytosis and degranulation, but they do not generate superoxide anion, nor do they kill catalase-positive organisms.

B False   Humoral immunity.

C False   Humoral immunity.

D True

E True   Leukocyte function.

Answer 82

A True

B True   The total haemolytic complement (CH50) is a useful screening technique for most diseases of complement system. This assay will not detect deficiencies of the alternative pathway components B, D and properdin.

C True   C1q, C1r, C1rs, C3, C4 and C2 are all associated with SLE-like syndrome (vasculitis).

D True   As well as C5, C6, C7 or C8 deficiency may be associated with recurrent neisserial infection.

E False   Deficiency of C1 esterase inhibitor is associated with hereditary angio-oedema.

Answer 83

A True   Associated with SLE, HIV, leukaemia and lymphoma.

B True   As in nephrotic syndrome.

C True

D True   As in SLE.

E False   It may occur after chemotherapy for malignancy.

Answer 84

A False Paediatric acquired immune deficiency syndrome (AIDS) is caused by human immunodeficiency virus type I. HIV-1 infects CD4+ T-lymphocytes, leading to immunodeficiency.

B False Blood products, sexual transmission and perinatal transmission.

C False Not generalised persistent lymphadenopathy.

D True

E True

Answer 85

A False CD4 depletion results in immunodeficiency.

B True

C True

D False

E True

Answer 86

A True HIV infection can be detected only after 6 months of age by commercial enzyme-linked immunoadsorbent assay and quantified by Western blots that measure antibody to specific viral polypeptides.

B True This is the most sensitive test to detect HIV-1 nucleic acid sequences and direct virus isolation from peripheral blood.

C True Hypergammaglobulinaemia is usually found.

D False It is the CD4:CD8 ratio that is reduced.

E False Other tests include P24 protein assay.

Answer 87

A True Increases cyclic AMP, generation of prostaglandins, vein permeability, pruritus, nasal mucus production and bronchial irritation.

B False Augments inactivation of histamine.

C False Neutrophil deactivation, aggregation and enzyme release.

D True Bronchodilation, relaxation of smooth muscle and rhinorrhoea.

E False Platelet aggregation, constriction of microvasculature and bronchoconstriction.

Answer 88

A False Lesions reach maximal size at 6–12 hours and disappear in 24–72 hours. The reaction is mediated by IgE.

B True

C False C4 and C3 can be involved in IgE-mediated reactions.

D True Serotonin is a vasoactive amine. It induces contraction of smooth muscle and increases vascular permeability.

E False Type II hypersensitivity reactions consist of a cytotoxic interaction between antigen and antibody at the cell surface involving IgG and IgM.

Answer 89

A True

B True

C True

D True

E True

Answer 90

A False The positive intradermal reaction is a weal of at least 5 mm of induration with surrounding erythema, occurring 15 minutes after injection of antigen.

B True This is associated with burning, pruritus, and doubling in size.

C True

D False This is an indication that the patient will necessarily have clinical symptoms on exposure to the allergen.

E False Daily or alternate day corticosteroid use for as long as one year may affect the release of histamine from the mast cells.

Answer 91

A False The Rast test is convenient and causes less patient anxiety. It is expensive and semiquantitative.

B False The skin test is very sensitive, is affected by antihistamine and dermatitis, has a broad selection of antigens, gives immediate results, is not expensive, and is sensitive to allergens.

C True

D False

E True

Answer 92

A True As well as antihistamines, sodium cromoglycate.

B True

C True

D True

E True Antiragweed IgE and IgG.

Answer 93

A True   After the first 3 days of life, the T wave is inverted in V4R and
          V1 and usually inverted in V2 and V3 in early childhood.
          Inverted T wave is normally seen in aVR and lead III.
          Pathological inverted T wave is associated with ventricular
          hypertrophy, myocardial disease, pericarditis and severe
          hypothyroidism. Flat T wave is seen in myocarditis and
          hypothyroidism while tall T wave is seen in hyperkalaemia.

B True

C False   The P wave absent in VF and may be seen with SVT.

D False   The heart rate is usually above 220/minute.

E False

Answer 94

A True

B False   This may lead to ventricular fibrillation and sudden death.

C False   Approximately 70–80% of patients with SVT have a normal
          heart.

D False   This is type B WPW. Type A is accessory pathway from left
          atrium to left ventricle.

E True

Answer 95

A True

B True   No other treatment is required.

C True   Surgery is not required unless the pulmonary pressure is
          nearer to systemic pressure, or the patient is suffering from
          failure to thrive and the hole is not getting smaller.

D False   Patients with a high flow of blood entering the pulmonary
          circuit at systemic pressure are those who will develop
          pulmonary vascular disease; it is in this group that surgery is
          most likely to be required.

E False   Prophylactic antibiotics are recommended in all types of VSD
          prior to any surgery.

Answer 96

A True This is due to increased flow of blood through the tricuspid valve. This murmur increases with inspiration and fades with expiration.

B True

C True Correction by umbrella or surgery is usually advised at an early age, at 2–3 years.

D True P–R interval is prolonged and absence of rsR in lead V4R and V1.

E False

Answer 97

A False In utero the ductus serves to divert blood from the lungs to descending aorta.

B True This is because the pressures in the aorta are higher than those in the pulmonary artery throughout the cardiac cycle.

C True

D False The pulse pressure is increased.

E False Functionally closes within 10–15 hours of birth.

Answer 98

A True The incidence is 5–7%.

B True This occurs only when there is collateral circulation between the aorta proximal and distal to the coarctation.

C False There is usually no murmur in newborn babies, but in children short systolic murmurs can be heard.

D True

E False In the newborn there is usually marked RVH, and LVH occurs in infancy and childhood.

Answer 99

A False

B True

C True During squatting, the arterial blood flow to the legs is reduced and this helps to maintain the systemic resistance so that more blood enters the lungs.

D True Surgical correction usually depends on the severity of the lesion, the type of anatomy and the size of the child.

E True These are usually given during cyanotic attacks. Patients should be warned about early morning hypoglycaemia.

Answer 100

A True

B True

C True

D True

E False

Answer 101
A False   In TGA without a VSD the baby usually looks healthy at birth but will develop cyanosis within the first 24 hours of life. There is no murmur and no heart failure will develop.

B False

C True

D False   The aorta is in front of and parallel with the pulmonary artery rather than crossing it as in the normal heart. This gives the "cottage-loaf" appearance of the heart on CXR.

E True   The lungs are not oligaemic.

Answer 102
A False   To the right ventricle below the annulus fibrosus.

B True   Especially in lead 2 as well as prolonged P–R interval, RBBB (complete or incomplete).

C True   The pulse has a small volume and the venous pulse may show prominent a or v waves. A systolic murmur can be heard at the left sternal edge as can three or four heart sounds. A characteristic scratchy diastolic murmur is usually present, best heard at the lower left sternal edge.

D False   As pulmonary resistance drops.

E True

Answer 103
A False   It usually occurs very late.

B True   Occurs especially during feeding and can be seen on scalp and face.

C True   If liver is enlarged more than 2 cm, it is a very valuable sign of heart failure.

D False   Not very good sign, except in older children.

E True   Gallop rhythm, tachypnoea, cardiomegaly, cough and restlessness.

Answer 104
A True   Oral high dose of amoxycillin 1 hour before dental treatment which will give minimal bactericidal levels for at least 10 hours.

B True   If child requires anaesthesia then amoxycillin can be given IM prior to surgery.

C True   Also patients with a prosthetic heart valve.

D False

E False

Answer 105
A True   Only during the acute phase of heart failure.
B False   The infant or child is breathless and NGT will help.
C False   The most important thing is to determine the cause. Diuretics are the first line of treatment, and digoxin is only needed if the patient deteriorates. Vasodilators have also been used to lower the systemic resistance and remove load from the left ventricle.
D True
E False   Hypokalaemia.

Answer 106
A True
B True
C True
D False   There is currently no vaccine against streptococcal bacterial infection.
E True   Long-term prophylaxis (Penicillin V) gives about 80% protection against further attacks of rheumatic fever.

Answer 107
A True   Early signs of bacterial endocarditis are fever, malaise, lassitude, loss of appetite and pallor due to anaemia.
B False
C True
D False
E False   This is a late manifestation, as are clubbing of the fingers and toes, heart failure, splinter haemorrhages, Osler's nodes and cerebral incidents.

Answer 108
A True
B True   It is within the normal range for this age group.
C True
D True
E False   Sodium nitroprusside and frusemide are more effective in hypertensive crises.

Answer 109
A True
B False   There is elevation of ST in all standard leads.
C False   It may develop.
D False
E True   Systemic lupus, rheumatoid disease, bacterial, viral and tuberculosis may all cause pericarditis.

Answer 110
A False By reducing heart rate, cardiac output and renin release.
B True Other features include agitation, confusion and depression.
C True
D True To reduce tremor.
E False Contraindicated, as in reactive airways and pulmonary insufficiency.

Answer 111
A True
B False
C True
D True Can lead to profound hypotension.
E False Vasoconstriction.

Answer 112
A True
B False It is within normal range.
C False The sum of S in V1 and R in V5 or V6 is >40 mm in children over 1 year of age, or >30 mm in those under 1 year of age.
D True Right atrial hypertrophy produces spiked P waves over 2.5 mm in leads 2 and V1 or V4R.
E True

Answer 113
A False ASD.
B False Not with PS; it may be associated with a large VSD or severe aortic stenosis.
C False ASD.
D True
E False Both PS and ASD.

Answer 114
A True
B False This is a serious problem. The cause must be found and treated.
C False It may cause death due to ventricular arrhythmia. Increased Q–T interval is seen in myocarditis, hypothyroidism, hypothermia and hypocalcaemia. It may be familial or associated with Lange–Nielsen syndrome.
D True It may also follow heart surgery.
E True Complete heart block.

Answer 115

A True   PDA, subclavian anomaly.

B False   Associated with dilatation of aorta and aneurysm of AO, also MI and mitral valve prolapse.

C False   Associated with supravalvular aortic stenosis and PS.

D True   Also VSD, ASD.

E True   Will also have small atrium.

Answer 116

A True   It is one of the glycogen storage diseases and has a very poor prognosis.

B False   Cardiomyopathy.

C True   Also fibrosis.

D True   Atherosclerosis associated with progeria.

E False   No cardiac problem.

Answer 117

A True

B True After birth, pulmonary vascular resistance declines rapidly as a consequence of vasodilatation due to gas filling the lungs, a rise in postnatal PO_2, reduction in PCO_2, increased pH, and release of vasoactive substance.

C False Usually occurs by a few hours after birth.

D True

E True

Answer 118

A True Also psychogenic.

B False

C True Mostly psychogenic.

D False May occur with DKA.

E True May also occur with other causes of metabolic acidosis such as RTA, CRF, low GFR, shock and inherited aminoaciduria.

Answer 119

A False Tachycardia is usually due to nebulised or IV bronchodilators.

B True Not very good in life-threatening asthma attack.

C False

D True Intercostal/subcostal recession and tracheal tug are all very good markers for the severity of asthma attack.

E True Fall in RR is a very poor prognostic sign and immediate intervention is required.

Answer 120

A True

B False

C True As well as by the PO_2 of the inspired gas, the haemoglobin oxygen capacity, and the respective alveolar gas and capillary blood flow in the lungs.

D False Angiotensin I is converted to angiotensin II in one passage through the pulmonary circulation. Some other vasoactive substances, e.g. serotonin, bradykinin, ATP, and prostaglandins E1, E2, and F2, are almost completely removed or inactivated by one passage through the pulmonary circulation.

E False It is directly proportional to CO_2 production and inversely proportional to alveolar ventilation.

Answer 121

A True

B True   Due to increase of haemoglobin level, red blood cells and blood volume.

C True   Due to decrease in the oxygen-binding capacity of haemoglobin. The arterial PO_2 is normal.

D True   Due to hypoxia and low Hb.

E True   Lung diseases cause inflammation, collapse, and fluid accumulation in alveoli which causes right to left shunt due to increased right-sided pressure.

Answer 122

A True

B False   Associated with both. Common with acute lung diseases or those of upper respiratory tract.

C True   Patients are usually tachypnoeic, cyanotic and use accessory muscles.

D True   Also with hypoxia and cardiac arrhythmias, renal failure and malnutrition.

E False

Answer 123

A False

B False

C True

D True

E True   Appear later.

Answer 124

A True

B False   The lesions are painful indurated red, hot, shiny, ovoid nodules. They are distributed almost symmetrically over the shins but may also occur on the calves, thighs, buttocks and upper extremities.

C True   May also be due to sarcoidosis, leptospirosis, cat-scratch disease, EBV, tularaemia, histoplasmosis, and Yersinia as well as drugs, e.g. sulphonamide and contraceptive pills.

D False

E False

Answer 125

A True   It usually occurs following increased intracranial pressure due to cerebral oedema.

B True

C True   Which may cause ICP and brain herniation.

D True

E False   Treat the cause with oxygenation.

Answer 126

A True
B True
C False   To the opposite side as well as pleural effusion.
D False   Usually respiratory distress, retraction and reduced air entry on the affected side.
E False   Pulsus paradoxus.

Answer 127

A False   pH is normal, especially in chronic lung diseases with healthy kidneys.
B False   Plasma bicarbonate level is high, as acidosis and high PCO_2 stimulate the kidney to increase hydrogen ion excretion as ammonium and tetratable acid and to generate and reabsorb more bicarbonate.
C True
D True
E True

Answer 128

A True   Due to hypoalbuminaemia.
B True   Due to malabsorption.
C True   These may cause nasal obstruction and rhinorrhoea.
D True   This is relatively frequent; 30% of newborn babies with CF may present with meconium ileus as first presentation.
E False

Answer 129

A True
B False   Liver diseases associated with CF are biliary cirrhosis, portal hypertension, obstructive jaundice and, rarely, biliary cirrhosis.
C True   This may develop in 2–5% of patients with CF.
D True   This is improved by controlling lung infection.
E True   Patients with CF should have glycosylated haemoglobin level checked annually.

Answer 130

A False   May interfere with growth, discolour teeth and cause pseudotumour cerebri in infants. It should only be used in children over 8 years of age.
B True   Other effects include optic neuritis, pellagra, hypersensitivity, SLE-like disease and hyperglycaemia.
C False   Thrombocytopenia, peripheral neuritis and optic neuritis are the commonest side effects.
D False   Hepatotoxicity, sideroblastic anaemia and urticaria.
E False

Answer 131

A True   It is also called hydrothorax. The fluid has a specific gravity of 1.015 and contains little protein and few cells. It may also be caused by venous obstruction by neoplasms, large lymph nodes and adhesions.

B True

C True   This can cause chylothorax by obstructing the thoracic duct, or be due to restrictive lung diseases, thrombosis of the duct or the subclavian vein.

D True

E True

Answer 132

A False   Occurs in both.

B False   Occurs in both.

C True   Also high fever, sore throat, dyspnoea and rapidly progressive respiratory obstruction.

D True

E False   Occurs in both.

Answer 133

A True   May be due to gastro-oesophageal reflux.

B True   As a source of recurrent infection.

C True   Such as house dust mites, smoking, pets or asthma.

D True

E True

Answer 134

A True   Hypoxia is universal but response to oxygen therapy is variable; it is usually not responsive to 100% oxygen.

B True   It is due to persistent right to left shunt via patent ductus arteriosus and foramen ovale after birth.

C True   There is usually profound hypoxia with normal or elevated PCO_2.

D False

E True   Other causes such as hypoglycaemia, HIE, meconium aspiration, pneumonia, group B streptococcal infection, HMD, and pulmonary hypoplasia should be excluded.

Answer 135

A True 95% of males are azoospermic due to failure of development of wolffian duct structures.

B False This occurs in only 2–3% of patients; biliary colic secondary to cholelithiasis may occur in the second decade of life.

C True There are 400 gene mutations that contribute to CF, occurring at a single locus on the long arm of chromosome 7.

D False Occurs in only 10–15% and more than 30% of siblings born subsequent to a child with meconium ileus.

E True

Answer 136

A False A significant proportion of infants with bronchiolitis have hyperactive airway during later childhood, especially those with a family history of atopy and exposure to smoking.

B True

C False It is very expensive and used in selected cases.

D False Nursing care, feeding and oxygen supplementation are the main therapeutic approaches for infants with acute bronchiolitis.

E False Corticosteroids have proved to be ineffective in this condition.

Gastroenterology answers

Answer 137
A True
B True
C True
D False
E True

Answer 138
A True   About 98% of natural fat is triglycerides. Triglycerides are hydrolysed in the duodenum by pancreatic lipase to monoglycerides and fatty acids and, with bile salts, form micelles, increasing fat solubility.

B False   To fatty acids and monoglycerides.

C True

D True   As well as monoglycerides.

E True   After re-esterification of fatty acids and monoglycerides to triglycerides, which are then coated by lipoproteins to form the chylomicrons, in which they are transported to the venous circulation via the lymph system and through the thoracic duct.

Answer 139
A True   As are oesophageal stricture due to corrosive ingestion, trauma, and chronic severe oesophagitis.

B False   Causes refusal to eat or drink because of pain.

C False

D False   Oesophageal atresia should be suspected in cases of maternal polyhydramnios, when a nasogastric tube cannot be passed after birth, if the neonate has excessive oral secretions, or if there is choking, cyanosis or coughing when feeding is attempted.

E True   Other neuromuscular disorders which may cause dysphagia are cerebral palsy, dermatomyositis, familial dysautonomia, scleroderma, Werdnig–Hoffmann disease and muscular dystrophy.

Answer 140
A False

B True   As well as idiopathic, which can cause frequent drop in lower oesophageal sphincter pressure.

C False

D True   Also Down's syndrome or any condition causing severe developmental delay.

E False

Answer 141
A True It is also associated with vitamin B_{12} deficiency, low serum iron and ferritin levels, allergy or toxic drug reaction, and trauma.

B False

C True

D False Recurrent herpes infection or any other viral infection does not usually cause aphthous ulcers as the lesions are localised to the mucocutaneous junction.

E True Mainly due to stress.

Answer 142
A True Offspring of a mother and, to a lesser extent, a father who had pyloric stenosis are at higher risk for pyloric stenosis (20%, 10% respectively).

B True As early as one week of age and up to 5 months of age.

C False Usually immediately after a feed. May be not projectile initially but subsequently becomes projectile.

D True

E False It is one of the manifestations, as is projectile vomiting. The presence of a pyloric mass can establish the diagnosis; abdominal ultrasound is a helpful diagnostic procedure.

Answer 143
A True

B False Rare.

C True Overfeeding, gastroenteritis, anatomical obstruction, toxic ingestion and medication are also common causes of vomiting in children.

D True Or milk allergy.

E True

Answer 144
A False May present with chronic diarrhoea, but with normal growth and general health.

B True Gluten enteropathy, lactase deficiency, cystic fibrosis, short gut, lymphangiectasia, congenital chloridorrhoea, abetalipoproteinaemia and inflammatory bowel diseases are other causes of chronic diarrhoea, malabsorption and abnormal growth.

C True

D True

E True

Answer 145

A True

B False   Asthma may cause failure to thrive but it is not a common cause.

C True   Conditions causing malabsorption, chronic infection, chromosomal abnormalities, malignancy, and recurrent infection of tonsils are major common causes of FTT.

D False   Inborn error of metabolism is associated with FTT.

E False

Answer 146

A True

B True   As in lactose intolerance.

C True

D True   Epilepsy, angioneurotic oedema, porphyria, sickle cell crisis and lead poisoning are also nonspecific causes of recurrent abdominal pain in children.

E False   Anal itching and vulvitis in girls are the commonest presentations.

Answer 147

A True   The diagnosis can be made by a good history and full examination. Laboratory tests and imaging are of some help.

B True

C False   Fever is usually low grade unless perforation has occurred.

D True

E True

Answer 148

A True   Anorexia is common and is the main cause of weight loss.

B False   Stool is bulky. Pale, smelly and bulky stools are associated with CF.

C False   Symptoms may occur as soon as a gluten-containing diet is introduced.

D True   Infants with gluten-sensitive enteropathy are also irritable, clingy and unhappy.

E False   Organomegaly is not associated with gluten-sensitive enteropathy in children.

Answer 149

A True The child with intussusception may present with diarrhoea, colicky pain, restlessness and vomiting. A sausage-shaped mass may be palpated in the right upper quadrant. Abdominal X-ray will show absence of gas in the caecum and ascending colon, and distended loops of intestine with fluid levels.

B False

C True Occurs uncommonly.

D True May also associated with metastatic tumours, parasitic infection and haemangioma.

E False Rectal prolapse may be associated with cystic fibrosis, malnutrition, acute diarrhoea, ulcerative colitis, pertussis or intestinal parasites. May also be idiopathic.

Answer 150

A False Biopsy in ulcerative colitis will show inflammation of crypts, crypt abscesses, oedema, mucosal depletion, foci of acute inflammatory cells and branching crypts.

B True Highly characteristic.

C False Ulcerative colitis.

D False Ulcerative colitis.

E True Non-caseating granulomas, fissures and full thickness involvement are associated with Crohn's disease.

Answer 151

A True This pain is relieved by vomiting and localised to the epigastrium or periumbilical area.

B False Upper and lower gastrointestinal tract obstruction can cause constipation.

C True As in duodenal and oesophageal atresia.

D False Is reduced or absent.

E True Copious in volume and frequent, with little abdominal distension.

Answer 152

A True

B True

C True By the seventh to eighth week in the human foetus.

D False Phenylalanine, tyrosine, methionine and tryptophan are increased.

E True

Answer 153

A False   From foetal haemoglobin (HbF).
B False   It is mostly unconjugated.
C True
D True   Also in conjugation.
E False   Both are primary bile acids. Deoxycholate and lithocholate are secondary bile acids.

Answer 154

A False   Conjugated.
B True
C True
D True
E True

Answer 155

A False   It is increased, but the diagnosis can be suspected in a previously healthy child who presents with a history of a viral-like illness followed by normal recovery. This is then followed by abrupt vomiting, lethargy, confusion and light coma that may progress to coma, decerebrate rigidity and flaccidity.
B True   ICP secondary to cerebral oedema is the major lethal factor. There are also high liver enzymes, coagulation abnormalities and hypoglycaemia.
C True
D False   The prodromal febrile illness is a URTI in 90% of cases, chicken pox in 5–7%.
E True   The liver is yellow or white due to high content of triglycerides.

Answer 156

A True
B True   This may follow in HBsAg-positive patients, as may vasculitis and arthritis.
C True   Coombs-positive anaemia and rash are common in patients with autoimmune chronic active hepatitis.
D True
E False   "Cushingoid features" may occur.

Answer 157

A True
B True
C True
D False   It is a benign condition.
E True

Answer 158

A True   The serum copper is elevated in early Wilson's disease; urinary copper excretion is increased.

B True   Also behavioural problems

C False Hepatic copper is increased on liver biopsy but is not diagnostic.

D True   D-penicillamine and triethylene tetramine dihydrochloride are also the primary chelating agents in treatment of Wilson's disease.

E False Chelation with D-penicillamine can increase urinary copper excretion, which can be of added value in the diagnosis of Wilson's disease.

Answer 159

A True   Also jaundice and encephalopathy due to liver failure.

B True   Gastrointestinal bleeding and splenomegaly are consistent features of portal hypertension.

C False

D True   Bleeding from oesophageal varices is the commonest presentation of portal hypertension.

E True

Answer 160

A False It increases the hydrostatic pressure.

B False More fluid enters the lymphatic system and weeps from liver.

C False It increases water absorption by kidneys.

D True   Also aldosterone, which leads to Na retention.

E True

Answer 161

A True   Storage disease.

B False

C True

D True   Iron overload.

E True

Metabolic disorder answers

Answer 162

A True Typical manifestations are glucosuria and ketonuria; random glucose is >6 mmol/l.

B False

C True Also -DR3, -BW15, and -DR4, located on chromosome 6.

D True Polyuria, polydipsia, polyphagia and weight loss constitute the classical presentation of diabetes in children.

E False

Answer 163

A True

B True The Somogyi phenomenon can be defined as hypoglycaemic episodes, which may be mild and manifest as late nocturnal or early morning sweating, night terrors, and headaches leading rapidly within 3–4 hours to ketosis, hyperglycaemia, ketonuria and excessive glucosuria.

C False The association between these two conditions is high.

D True Also ketosis and hyperglycaemia.

E False 10–20% of daily insulin dose as short-acting insulin can be added.

Answer 164

A False Ketones are high because of incomplete utilisation of fat.

B True

C True

D False It may be normal, especially during a fasting period.

E True

Answer 165

A True

B True

C False Serum osmolality is usually normal.

D True The bicarbonate is <15 mmol/l and pH <7.20.

E False It is helpful but laboratory plasma glucose is the confirmatory test.

Answer 166

A True
B False No loading dose of insulin is needed and the dose is 0.025–0.1 u/kg/day as infusion.
C True
D True When the acidosis is corrected and the patient is rehydrated.
E False It can be given in severe acidosis, when there is deterioration of GCS or ventilation is required. Most important is fluid replacement and insulin infusion, which will help to correct acidosis very slowly over the first 24 hours.

Answer 167

A True Sequelae are most likely in an infant with hyperinsulinaemia and severe recurrent hypoglycaemia, especially if this is accompanied by hypoxia.
B True
C True Common features of hypoglycaemia are anxiety, tachycardia, headaches, mental confusion, visual disturbances, organic personality changes, inability to concentrate, and possibly seizures.
D False
E False

Answer 168

A True
B False May cause hypoglycaemia.
C True As emergency treatment.
D True As well as corticosteroids and glucose at a dose of 2–5 ml/kg of 10% as emergency treatment. This is followed by continuous glucose infusion at 6–8 mg/kg/min.
E False

Answer 169

A False Von Gierke's disease (GSDla) is associated with deficiency of glucose-6-phosphatase. This is associated with hypoglycaemia, lactic acidosis, hyperuricacidaemia, gout and bleeding. The galactose and fructose are not converted to glucose; this test can be used but may precipitate acidosis.

B False It is phenylalanine hydroxylase.

C True

D False Purine nucleoside phosphorylase deficiency is associated with deficiency of cellular immunity. Lesch–Nyhan syndrome is associated with hypoxanthine guanine phosphoribosyl transferase deficiency; it presents as early motor developmental delay and later with extrapyramidal choreoathetoid movements, hyper-reflexia, ankle clonus and spasticity with compulsive self-destructive behaviour.

E True

Answer 170

A True

B True

C False It is inherited as an X-linked recessive trait with clinical features of coarse facial features, short stature, joint stiffness, hepatosplenomegaly and hernias. Mental retardation is severe and hearing loss is common.

D False Inherited as autosomal recessive.

E True Tyrosinaemia type I presents in two forms: (1) at the age of 6 months with FTT, developmental delay, jaundice, hepatomegaly, hypoglycaemia, vomiting, diarrhoea and bleeding tendencies; (2) in chronic form, which may present after the first birthday with FTT, developmental delay, cirrhosis, RTA and rickets.

Answer 171

A True Also gout, bleeding tendencies, no rise of blood glucose after subcutaneous adrenaline or glucagon with normal catecholamine production.

B True

C True

D True No involvement of skeletal or cardiac muscle, leukocytes or skin fibroblasts.

E True

Answer 172

A True The clinical manifestations of fatty oxidation defect (medium chain acyl-CoA-dehydrogenase deficiency) are hypoglycaemia, low plasma and urinary ketones, abnormal LFT, urate, urea, high ammonia with prolonged TT and PTT. The diagnosis can be made by obtaining fasting urinary organic acid which will show low concentration of medium-chain dicarboxylic acid by gas chromatography–mass spectroscopy.

B False

C True Liver biopsy during acute illness shows increased triglyceride deposition.

D True

E True

Answer 173

A False Fructose 1,6 diphosphatase aldolase deficiency is the commonest enzyme deficiency.

B True

C False In hypoglycaemia and progressive liver disease, a fructose tolerance test is contraindicated because it may be followed by hypoglycaemia, shock and death.

D True Clinical features usually appear when there is ingestion of fructose-containing foods.

E False Ammonia level is usually normal in patients with fructosaemia. Urine-reducing substances may show fructose by chromatography.

Answer 174

A True It is due to lipoprotein lipase deficiency and is very rare with massively high level of triglycerides.

B False It is inherited as autosomal dominant and characterised by xanthoma striata palmaris. Coronary heart disease and peripheral vascular disease are common.

C True It is the most common form of hyperlipidaemia with high cholesterol level of >300 mg/dl, familial history of myocardial infarction and tendon xanthomas. The gene has been mapped to chromosome 19 with a defect in the LDL receptor.

D True It is associated with high level of chylomicrons and VLDL triglycerides.

E False This is associated with Type I.

Answer 175

A True   Heme is composed of ferrous iron and protoporphyrin and is essential for life.

B False   It may present with abdominal pain, nausea, constipation, vomiting and urinary retention.

C True

D False   It is an early manifestation of congenital erythropoietic porphyria.

E True   The clinical manifestation of hereditary coproporphyria is abdominal pain. Neurological and psychiatric manifestations are also common.

Answer 176

A False   The majority presented in the first few days of life.

B True   It is associated with poor feeding, lethargy which may progress to deep coma, and death. Myoclonic seizures and hiccups are common.

C True   Severe hyperglycinaemia and hyperglycinuria is common.

D False   Sodium valproate is a cause of moderate rise in serum and CSF glycine in epileptic patients.

E True   In 80% of patients; the rest have a T protein defect.

Endocrinology answers

Answer 177

A True
B True
C False   It is a synthetic analogue of vasopressin.
D True   Also milk production.
E False   Pharmacological quantities have a pressor effect.

Answer 178

A False
B True   Any lesion causing damage to the neurohypophyseal unit will cause diabetes insipidus. Craniopharyngioma, optic glioma, and germinoma are the tumours that most commonly cause DI. About 25% of patients with histiocytosis may develop DI. It can also be inherited as autosomal dominant. It is associated with Wolfram syndrome (DIDMOD). In 20% it is idiopathic.

C False
D True
E True

Answer 179

A True
B False   Total daily urinary sodium excretion is normal in central DI. The daily volume of urine may exceed 4–10 litres with a specific gravity of 1.001–1.005, and urine osmolality of 50–200 mOsm/kg water.

C True
D True   Urine osmolality that is greater after a period of dehydration than after administration of DDAVP indicates that patients can produce vasopressin. The diagnosis of compulsive water drinking can be made if patients fail to produce a concentrated urine when fluids are withheld.

E False   It is not effective and not recommended orally.

Answer 180

A False   It increases glucose uptake by muscles.
B True
C True
D True
E False   It decreases rather than increases adipose tissue lipids.

Answer 181

A True   Other common forms of presentation include obesity, striae, pubertal developmental delay, weakness, headache and deterioration in school performance.

B True

C True

D True   Most prominent in the spine.

E True   Laboratory findings of polycythaemia, lymphopenia and eosinopenia are common. The normal serum cortisol is elevated at 8 am and decreased to less than 5% by 8 pm. This normal diurnal rhythm is lost in patients with Cushing's syndrome. The cortisol level is elevated at 8 pm. Other electrolytes are normal.

Answer 182

A True   Anencephaly, holoprosencephaly and septo-optic dysplasia are associated with growth hormone deficiency. Optic nerve dysplasia, Turner's, Russell–Silver, Rieger's, Williams' and CHARGE syndrome may also be associated with hypopituitarism.

B True

C False   IGF-1 receptor defect may cause GH deficiency.

D True

E False   This follows severe septicaemia, as in meningococcal sepsis.

Answer 183

A True

B False   Hyperinsulinism may cause obesity. Insulin decreases lipolysis and increases fat synthesis and uptake. The obese person becomes resistant to insulin, which results in an increase in insulin levels in blood.

C True   Other syndromes associated with obesity include Cushing's, Stein–Leventhal (polycystic ovary), Turner's, Cohen's, Carpenter's and Alstrom–Hallgren syndromes.

D False

E True

Answer 184

A True   The salt-losing variant is associated with progressive weight loss, dehydration, vomiting, anorexia and virilisation in females.

B False

C True   Serum sodium and chloride are low, with high levels of potassium and renin. The 17-hydroxyprogesterone level is markedly high and there is a high level of urinary 17-ketosteroids and pregnanetriol.

D False   This is associated with 11β-hydroxylase defect.

E True

Answer 185

A True Most infants die in early infancy as adrenal steroids usually fail to become elevated.

B True

C False This is characterised by hypertension, hypokalaemia and suppression of renin and aldosterone production. Male virilisation is not completed, presenting as phenotypic females or pseudohermaphroditism. Affected females usually present with failure to develop sexual characteristics at the expected time of puberty.

E True There is no difference between males and females.

E False This occurs in 5% of patients with adrenal hyperplasia. The elevated levels of deoxycortisol (DOC) are thought to cause the hypertension and prevent symptoms of salt loss. The plasma level of 11-deoxycortisol and DOC is elevated.

Answer 186

A True

B False In salt-losing cases, oral hydrocortisone, 9α-fluorocortisol and sodium chloride are the recommended treatment. In non-salt-losing cases, hydrocortisone is required; 9α-fluorocortisol is required only if the renin level is high.

C False If the child is more than 10% dehydrated, normal saline is needed, then calculate fluid over 24 hours (maintenance plus deficit).

D False Short stature.

E False Occurs in both sexes.

Answer 187

A True As with side effects of steroids.

B True

C True

D False This may happen if glucocorticoids are stopped suddenly.

E True

Answer 188

A True Type 1 autoimmune polyendocrinopathy is associated with mucocutaneous candidiases, hypoparathyroidism, Addison's disease, gonadal failure, vitiligo, keratopathy, enamel hypoplasia, nail dystrophy, intestinal malabsorption and chronic hepatic failure. Hypothyroidism and IDDM occur in 105% of patients with type 1.

B True

C True

D False It is associated with autoimmune thyroid disease.

E False Hypoparathyroidism associated with type 1 autoimmune polyendocrinopathy.

Answer 189

A True
B False   It is not commonly associated with hypoaldosteronism.
C False   Hypertension is invariably associated with hyperaldosteronism.
D False   Hyperkalaemia, hyperchloraemia and acidosis are common features. Salt loss is common and plasma renin is elevated.
E False   Subtotal adrenalectomy rather than total is required.

Answer 190

A True
B False   The total urinary excretion of catecholamines usually exceeds 300 mcg/day.
C True   VMA is the major metabolite of epinephrine, norepinephrine, and metanephrine.
D False   It is mainly norepinephrine.
E False   Chromaffin cells can be found along the abdominal sympathetic chain.

Answer 191

A False   Development usually starts between the 4th and 6th weeks of foetal life.
B True   The gene is usually on the short arm of the Y chromosome.
C True
D False   Sertoli cells can produce anti-mullerian hormone which inhibits mullerian duct development.
E True

Answer 192

A True   They are usually stored as thyroglobulin in the lumen of the follicle.
B True   This is by activation of proteases and peptidases to release T3 and T4 from thyroglobulin.
C False   Only 20% is secreted by the thyroid gland; the rest is produced by deiodination of T4 in the liver, kidney and other peripheral tissues.
D False   T3 and T4 do not cross the placenta.
E False

Answer 193

A False   School work is usually not affected.

B True   This is the first clinical feature. It may be associated with others such as constipation, cold intolerance, decreased energy and excessive sleep. Osseous maturation is delayed.

C True

D True   Myxoedematous change of the skin is a common feature which develops later.

E False   This is associated with the adult type.

Answer 194

A False   It is familial.

B False   It is characterised histologically by lymphocytic infiltration of the thyroid gland. The serum antibody for thyroid peroxidase is positive in most patients and the antiglobulin test for thyroid antibodies is positive in 50% of patients.

C True   The TSH level is moderately high in some euthyroid patients.

D True   Most are euthyroid, and some have signs of hypothyroidism.

E True   Goitre usually persists for years.

Answer 195

A False   Hypocalcaemia, hyperphosphataemia, normal serum alkaline phosphatase, low 1,25(OH)2D3, and normal magnesium serum level.

B True

C True

D True   Muscular pain, cramps, numbness, stiffness, tingling of hand and feet, positive Chvostek or Trousseau sign, and convulsions. These features of hypoparathyroidism may be the presenting features.

E False

Haematology answers

Answer 196

A True   This is inherited as an autosomal dominant trait with no significant clinical features. Iron, folic acid and vitamin B_{12} deficiency may cause elliptocytosis.

B False   Reticulocytes are diminished even when it is severe.

C True   All types of haemolytic anaemia are associated with reticulocytosis.

D False

E True

Answer 197

A True   Leukaemoid reaction is associated with diabetic ketoacidosis and hepatic failure.

B True   Sepsis, azotaemia and malignancy involving bone marrow.

C True

D True

E True

Answer 198

A False   Platelet count and prothrombin time are normal; bleeding time is prolonged.

B False   The platelets in von Willebrand's disease have decreased adhesiveness and do not aggregate when the antibiotic ristocetin is added to platelet-rich plasma.

C True

D True

E True

Answer 199

A False   Exocrine pancreatic dysfunction is associated with Schwachman syndrome.

B False   This is a feature of dyskeratosis congenita.

C True   Fanconi anaemia is associated with upper limb abnormalities, skin pigmentation, renal malformation, skeletal abnormalities and pancytopenia. The thumb is preserved in TAR syndrome.

D False   Both have not been fully studied. Androgens, bone marrow transplant and steroids are the current treatment in patients with Fanconi anaemia.

E False

Answer 200

A True   Schwachman syndrome is characterised by thoracic dystrophy, ichthyosis, diabetes mellitus, red cell hypoplasia, elevated HbF, metaphyseal dysplasia and psychomotor delay.

B False

C True

D True   With risk of malignancy and androgenisation in females.

E False

Answer 201

A True   It is characterised by severe neutropenia and frequent bacterial infection. It is inherited as autosomal recessive.

B False   It is pure red cell aplasia with anaemia as early as 2–3 months of age, dysmorphic facies or upper extremity defects.

C True   Haemolytic anaemia and pancytopenia are other features of this condition.

D True   Infection with this virus in utero may cause pure red cell aplasia in infancy.

E True

Answer 202

A False   It is an acute phase reaction which is increased in response to recent infection and gives false negative results.

B False   It is helpful but not diagnostic. The level of serum ferritin provides a relatively accurate estimate of body iron stores in the absence of inflammatory disease.

C False   It is helpful but not diagnostic.

D False   It is helpful but not diagnostic.

E True   In the absence of erythroid hyperplasia.

Answer 203

A False   Sideroblastic anaemia is characterised by hypochromic, microcytic anaemia due to abnormalities of heme metabolism. The serum iron level is increased. Acquired sideroblastic anaemia may be caused by chronic inflammatory diseases, malignancy and alcoholism.

B True

C True

D False

E False

Answer 204

A True Following regular transfusion.
B True Following regular transfusion and sickle cell crisis.
C True Secondary to haemolysis.
D True Secondary to haemolysis.
E True Secondary to haemolysis.

Answer 205

A False It is low with microcytic anaemia, and red blood cell distribution is normal.
B False It is low.
C True High ferritin is an acute phase reaction and it does not reflect iron deficiency anaemia.
D True
E False It is low.

Answer 206

A False It can be given if poor compliance is suspected, but should be avoided in the newborn.
B True There is a risk of iron overload as transferrin level is low.
C True As plasma transferrin level is reduced.
D False Can be given if follow-up is difficult, for example in rural areas.
E True

Answer 207

A True
B True
C True The other organs involved in polyendocrinopathy syndrome include adrenals, parathyroid, ovaries and thyroid.
D True
E True Also total and subtotal gastrectomy.

Answer 208

A True Haemolytic anaemia, surgical removal or small intestinal disorders, and infection may cause folic acid deficiency.
B True As with sodium valproate and phenytoin.
C True
D False Is not associated with any anaemia.
E False

Answer 209

A False Warm.
B False
C True As well as warm.
D False Warm.
E True

Answer 210

A True

B True

C True   Can also detect C3b, as in autoimmune haemolytic anaemia of warm and cold antibody.

D False   It is associated with autoimmune anaemia. This can be used in blood group and cross match. The positive indirect Coombs test is associated with autoimmune haemolytic anaemia (warm antibody).

E True

Answer 211

A True   Other drugs that can cause autoimmune haemolytic anaemia are quinine, quanidine, phenacetin and alpha aminobutyric acid.

B False

C True   Only in high doses.

D True

E False

Answer 212

A True   Other clinical features are aplastic, painful, avascular abdominal crises, acute chest syndrome, stroke, priapism, leg ulcers, enuresis, damage to renal tubules and eyes, iron deficiency and pneumococcal sepsis.

B True

C False   Gallbladder stones.

D True

E True

Answer 213

A False   IV fluid should be 150% of maintenance over 24 hours. Observe output.

B True

C False   Exchange transfusion is indicated when there is acute chest syndrome, stroke or a high percentage of sickle cells in acute haemolytic crisis.

D False   CXR may be indicated in chest pain or chest signs.

E False   Give oral analgesia, then change to IV morphine if pain score is high (>5).

Answer 214

A False   It is low.

B True

C True

D True

E True

Answer 215

A True   Microcytosis, target cells, Heinz bodies, high serum iron and bilirubin, and high foetal haemoglobin level are other features of thalassaemia.

B True

C False   There is a total or partial deletion of the globin chain gene and nucleotide substitutions, deletions or insertions. This will cause decrease or absence of mRNA of the globin chain, which suppresses the synthesis of the haemoglobin polypeptide chain.

D True

E False   It is usually manifested by the age of 4–6 months.

Answer 216

A False   Enzyme deficiency.

B True   Hereditary elliptocytosis, pyropoikilocytosis, stomatocytosis and paroxysmal nocturnal haemoglobinuria are other anaemias associated with a cell membrane defect.

C False   It is due to a globin chain synthesis defect.

D True

E True   Acanthocytosis.

Answer 217

A True

B True

C True

D True

E False

Answer 218

A True   Aplastic anaemia, Kostmann disease, Chediak–Higashi and Schwachman syndromes, cartilage–hair hypoplasia and AIDS are associated with neutropenia.

B False   Glycogen storage disease type Ib.

C True

D True

E True   Transient neutropenia as with viral, nutritional, drug-induced and neonatal sepsis.

Answer 219

A True

B False   Penicillin and nitrofurantoin can cause eosinophilia

C True

D False   Ulcerative colitis, JCA, iron deficiency and chronic renal failure are associated with basophilia.

E False   Tuberculosis, systemic mycosis, bacterial endocarditis, inflammatory bowel diseases and protozoan infections cause monocytosis.

Answer 220

A True Down's syndrome, Fanconi anaemia, Kostmann disease and Diamond–Blackfan anaemia are associated with increased risk of leukaemia.

B True

C False

D False Exposure to irradiation is a possible cause of leukaemia.

E True

Answer 221

A True The platelets are large and there is decreased ristocetin-induced platelet aggregation.

B True They are small.

C False They are normal.

D False Normal in shape.

E True

Nephrology answers

Answer 222

A False Sometimes need to be reduced.
B True   May increase by 10% for each 1C° above 37C°.
C True   The Na and Cl requirement is doubled in sick children with CF.
D False There is a risk of SIADH.
E True   The rate of metabolism is increased.

Answer 223

A True
B False This may happen in acute renal failure with low sodium.
C False It is also caused by gain of water in excess of sodium as in oedematous states, SIADH, renal failure, and excess water intake.
D True   This happens in children with constipation who are treated with clean prep.
E True

Answer 224

A False Cardiac failure will cause an increase in capillary blood pressure.
B True
C True
D False Increase in capillary permeability will cause oedema.
E False In burns there is an increase in oncotic pressure which increases the capillary permeability.

Answer 225

A False Fluid restriction as in fluid overload.
B True
C True
D True   Fluid restriction up to one-third of daily requirement in acute SIADH; intravenous loop diuretics can be used. Lithium is also used in treatment of chronic SIADH.
E False By fluid restriction.

Answer 226

A True

B False Iodogenic osmoles occur post treatment and may cause cerebral oedema.

C True Identification of the cause is most important before starting fluid. If dehydration is present due to any cause, 10 ml/kg of 0.9% NaCl should be given over one hour, then calculate the maintenance plus the deficit and give over 48 hours if there is no oliguria and over 72 hours if oliguria is present.

D True

E False It is not common but it may happen.

Answer 227

A True RTA and insulin therapy in DKA are other causes.

B False ECG changes associated with hyperkalaemia are T wave inversion, U wave exaggeration and bradyarrhythmias.

C False It should be 0.20–0.25 mmol/kg/h.

D False Potassium chloride is usually used in conditions with alkalotic states; in conditions associated with metabolic acidosis such as RTA, the citrate salt should be used.

E False Skeletal and cardiac muscle are also affected.

Answer 228

A True The first symptoms of post-streptococcal glomerulonephritis are facial swelling followed by swelling of feet and abdomen.

B True Gross haematuria occurs in 30–40% of patients.

C False

D True High blood pressure is present in the majority of patients, and 5% may develop hypertensive encephalopathy with convulsion and coma. Pallor is common due to oedema.

E True The C3 and C4 are low, ASO titres are high, urea and creatinine may be high or normal, proteinuria is present but not gross.

Answer 229

A True Highly concentrated urine, pyuria, bacteruria, phenazopyridine, and high levels of penicillin and cephalosporins are other reasons for false positive results being obtained by dipstick or protein precipitation methods.

B True

C False False negative.

D True

E False False negative. Also with diluted urine.

Answer 230

A True   As well as FSGS.
B False   This is associated with MPGN.
C False   Only a third of these patients respond to steroids.
D True   In only 10% of patients with MCNS.
E True

Answer 231

A False   In this age group, renal biopsy can be done if there is no response to steroids within a month of treatment.
B True
C False   Solitary kidney, bleeding disorders, severe azotaemia, uncontrolled hypertension, intrarenal malignancy, chronic renal failure, perinephric abscess, hydronephrosis, severe anaemia, marked obesity, nephrocalcinosis and pyelonephritis are contraindications for renal biopsy.
D False   This is commonly associated with MPGN or SLE.
E True

Answer 232

A True
B False   Congenital glomerulosclerosis, nail–patella syndrome, interstitial nephritis, infantile microcytic disease, diffuse, focal sclerosis and MCNS are causes of primary infantile nephrotic syndrome.
C True   Syphilis, CMV, Wilms' tumour, mercury toxicity, nephroblastoma and SLE can cause secondary infantile nephrotic syndrome.
D True
E False

Answer 233

A True   Tuberculosis, schistosomiasis, adenovirus, trauma, glomerulonephritis, hydronephrosis, diverticula, arteritis, kidney infarction, bleeding disorders, cyclophosphamide and exercise are the main causes of haematuria.
B True
C True
D True   In children.
E True

Answer 234

A True   It is autosomal recessive.
B False   Prune belly syndrome is associated with hydronephrosis; renal medullary dysplasia is associated with Beckwith–Wiedemann syndrome.
C True
D False   It is renal hypoplasia.
E True

Answer 235

A True
B False   This may cause unilateral enlargement.
C True
D False   Bilateral Wilms' tumour occurs in only 10% of patients.
E True

Answer 236

A True   Other causes include meatal ulcer, UTI, vulvovaginitis and acute nephritis.
B True   Other drugs that may cause dysuria are amitriptyline, chlordiazepoxide, sulphonamides, imipramine and cyclophosphamide.
C False
D False
E True   Also napkin dermatitis.

Answer 237

A False   It is secondary.
B True
C True
D False   SLE, Henoch–Schönlein purpura, scleroderma, mixed connective tissue diseases and vasculitis are causes of secondary glomerulonephritis.
E False

Answer 238

A False   This is the first drug to be given and it antagonises the effect of potassium.
B False   This can shift K into cells but does not remove it from the body.
C True   Haemodialysis for rapid removal or gradual removal by peritoneal dialysis.
D False   This is to shift potassium into cells.
E True

Answer 239

A False   This can be used as non-acute treatment.
B False   Insensible losses of 300 ml/m^2 of body surface area + fluid lost
is used as fluid therapy.
C True
D True
E False   400 kcal/m^2 of body surface area is used in ARF.

Answer 240

A True   Failure of fluid overload to respond to medical treatment,
symptomatic electrolyte disturbances such as hyponatraemia,
metabolic acidosis, hyperphosphataemia, hypocalcaemia,
hyperkalaemia and signs of uraemia are indications for dialysis.
B True
C False   Urea level is 50 mmol/l or more.
D True
E False

Answer 241

A True   It is also cheap and can be used while the patient is waiting for
a transplant in the short term.
B False   Haemodialysis.
C False   Is practically difficult.
D False   Haemodialysis.
E False   Haemodialysis.

Answer 242

A True   Hypokalaemia, polyuria, hypercalciuria, chronic acidosis and
inability to lower urine pH below 5.8 are features of distal
renal tubular acidosis.
B False
C False   Proximal RTA.
D False   Proximal RTA.
E False   Proximal RTA.

Answer 243

A True
B False   Hypokalaemia and hypocalcaemia can cause urine
concentrating defect.
C True
D True   This is via the urea-glucose osmotic effect.
E True

Answer 244

  A True   Trauma, surgery, calculus, glomerulonephritis, severe dehydration and cystitis may all lead to pyuria.

  B True

  C False

  D False

  E False

Answer 245

  A False   Distal RTA, idiopathic hypercalciuria, oxalosis and hypothyroidism can cause hypercalciuria and medullary nephrocalcinosis, but not hypercalcaemia.

  B True   Prolonged immobilisation and sarcoidosis are conditions which cause medullary nephrocalcinosis.

  C False

  D False

  E True

Neuroanatomy and neurophysiology answers

Answer 246
A False
B True
C False SI and S2 is tibial; L2,3,4 is femoral nerve.
D True
E True

Answer 247
A True
B False Musculocutaneous and median nerves.
C True
D True
E False Eleven only.

Answer 248
A True
B True
C False The superficial radial nerve supplies the extensor carpi radialis brevis, digitorum communis, carpi longus, pollicis brevis, indicis proprius, supinator and abductor pollicis longus.
D False Thumb, index and medial aspect of middle finger excluding terminal phalanges.
E True

Answer 249
A True
B True
C False From L2,3,4.
D False Innervated by the obturator nerve.
E False Adductor group innervated by the femoral nerve.

Answer 250
A True
B True Also jaw jerk and sneezing reflex.
C True
D True
E True

Answer 251
A True
B False   Amygdala.
C True
D False   Occipital lobe.
E True

Answer 252
A True
B True
C True
D False
E True

Answer 253
A True
B False
C True
D False
E True

Answer 254
A True
B False
C False
D True
E False

Answer 255
A False
B False
C False
D True
E True

Answer 256
A False   Arises from pons.
B True
C True
D False   Arises from midbrain.
E True

Answer 257

A True
B True
C True
D False
E False

Answer 258

A True
B True
C True
D True
E False

Answer 259

A True
B False
C True
D True
E True

Answer 260

A True
B True
C False
D True
E True

Answer 261

A False
B True
C True
D False
E True

Answer 262

A True
B False   The function of myelin and synaptic membrane is isolation.
C True
D False   The function of lysosomes is degrading reactions; that of the Golgi body is secretion.
E True

Answer 263

A True

B True

C True

D True

E False   The triceps reflex occurs by the radial nerve.

Answer 264

A False   It is also secreted by autonomic ganglia, parasympathetic neurones, motor nuclei of cranial nerves, caudate nucleus, basal nucleus of Meynert and portions of the limbic system.

B True   It is also secreted by the pineal gland and nucleus of Raphe.

C True   It is also found in the cerebellum, hippocampus and strionigral system.

D True   It is also secreted from the midbrain.

E False   Glutamic acid and glycine are found in spinal cord.

Answer 265

A True

B True

C True   As well as the buttocks, lateral aspect of legs, medial aspect of knees, soles of the feet and inguinal areas.

D True   The other three muscles are supplied by the lateral plantar nerve.

E True

Neurology answers

Answer 266

A True   It is inherited as X-linked recessive in 80%.
B True
C False   EMG is always abnormal with evidence of myopathy.
D True
E True   Can cause cardiomyopathy in the later stages.

Answer 267

A True   Also glossopharyngeal.
B False
C True
D False
E False

Answer 268

A False   Vertical gaze apraxia and no nystagmus.
B True   Is the most common cause (acquired and congenital).
C False   Vertical nystagmus as well as spinocerebellar degeneration.
D True   Is also associated with thiamine deficiency, phenytoin toxicity and hypomagnesaemia.
E False   Horizontal nystagmus.

Answer 269

A False   Characterised by abnormal sleep EEG.
B True   Other manifestations are generalised tonic/clonic seizures with aphasia and mouth turned to one side. Sleep EEG with centro-temporal spikes is diagnostic.
C True   Hypoglycaemia.
D True   Hypoglycaemia.
E False   Complex partial seizures, mainly when awake.

Answer 270

A True   HSV-2 causes the majority of encephalitis in the newborn, and HSV-1 at any age.
B True   As changes on CT may take longer to appear, MRI is more sensitive as an early neuroimaging test.
C True   Temporal lobe epilepsy.
D False   Leukocytosis, red cells, normal glucose and slightly raised protein.
E True   This is the minimum duration of treatment as relapse can occur, leading to high morbidity and mortality. Acyclovir should be given in the first 72 hours of the illness.

Answer 271
A False
B True
C True
D True
E False

Answer 272
A False   It affects mainly the proximal muscle groups with weakness, stiffness and pain.
B False   Only in adults.
C False   MRI will show evidence of myositis and is a good guide for muscle biopsy.
D False   Methotrexate, cyclosporine and azathioprine can be used in treatment.
E True

Answer 273
A False   Also occurs in girls.
B False   Carbamazepine will make it worse. Sodium valproate, lamotrigine and topiramate control seizure activity very well.
C False   Usually myoclonic absence or tonic/clonic or simple absence.
D True   Generalised poly spike discharges with clinical seizures and slow wave occurring afterwards.
E True

Answer 274
A True
B False   Ulnar nerve injury.
C False   Third and fourth by ulnar, and first and second by median.
D True
E False

Answer 275
A True
B True
C False   Gelastic seizures are associated with hypothalamic hamartoma.
D False   It is diagnostic in myoclonic absence seizures.
E True

Answer 276
A True
B False   Also unmyelinated.
C True
D False
E True

Answer 277

A True   Also multiple sclerosis. MRI will show increased signal on T2-weighted images of the white matter.

B True

C False   Cortical involvement (grey matter).

D False   Due to hypothalamic hamartoma.

E False   Atrophy of caudate nucleus and cerebral cortex on MRI.

Answer 278

A True   As well as angiokeratomas on the face, rhabdomyomas of kidney and heart.

B True   It is associated with cysts of kidney, bone and lung. Mental retardation and seizures are the other commonest clinical features.

C True   Periventricular calcification is common.

D False   Is a feature of neurofibromatosis type I.

E False   Radiological feature of Sturge–Weber syndrome.

Answer 279

A False   Small pupil.

B True   It is also called tonic pupil, which is associated with dysautonomia.

C True   As well as all ocular muscles except the lateral and medial rectus.

D False   Features include unilateral ptosis, miosis and anhidrosis of the face.

E True

Answer 280

A False

B True

C False

D True

E False

Answer 281

A True

B True

C True

D True

E False

Answer 282

A True Epilepsy is the most common manifestation and it is associated with partial seizures.

B True The earliest seizures are myoclonic (infantile spasms).

C True Focal or generalised seizures, infantile spasms may occur.

D True Focal seizures which are difficult to control.

E False It is associated with ocular and cutaneous symptoms with lesser neurological problems.

Answer 283

A False It is very good for generalised seizures as well as focal seizures.

B False Weight gain is one of the commonest side effects.

C False Can be given orally, rectally and intravenously.

D False

E False Can cause thinning of hair and hair loss. Other side effects including liver failure and polycystic ovary syndrome improve when treatment is stopped.

Answer 284

A False Intermittent ataxia with neurological deficit.

B True It is due to vasculitis.

C False Basilar artery migraine is one cause of intermittent ataxia with visual symptoms in which true seizures may occur.

D True True seizures may present as ataxia (epileptic pseudoataxia).

E True It is manifested as ophthalmoplegia.

Answer 285

A True As well as third and seventh nerve palsy.

B True Present in almost all cases.

C False Headache is the most common feature.

E False It is usually high and can be >40 mmHg.

E True After refeeding of malnourished child.

Answer 286

A True May be preceded by other manifestations of rheumatic fever.

B True Child becomes fidgety and clumsy with involuntary movements of various types.

C False The speech is dysarthritic and explosive.

D False That is a feature of tics.

E True Haloperidol is the classical treatment but sodium valproate can also be used.

Answer 287

A False   Both sides.
B True   Including CMV, HSV, hepatitis A and adenoviruses.
C True   Paraplegia, sphincter paralysis and marked sensory loss are the main clinical features. Back pain is observed in 60% of cases.
D True
E False   It is found in only half of patients.

Answer 288

A True
B False   This can be seen on cranial CT; MRI does not show calcification.
C True   This lesion is highly correlated with the complex partial seizures of temporal lobe origin.
D True
E False   This can be seen on cranial CT.

Answer 289

A False   Typical absence lasts only 5–15 seconds.
B False   Generalised seizures without a postictal phase.
C True
D False   EEG will show generalised rhythmical bursts of spike–wave complexes at 3 Hz with abrupt onset and termination.
E False   Eyes are open and the child stares.

Answer 290

A True   Visual hallucinations of colours and shapes.
B False   This symptom is associated with nocturnal seizures of occipital lobe epilepsy.
C True   It is called fixation-off phenomenon.
D True
E True   Most, if not all cases of occipital lobe epilepsy with this classification are associated with coeliac disease; the reason for this relationship is not understood.

Answer 291

A True
B True
C True
D False   Seizures appear within the first year of life.
E False   Skin manifestations may appear at birth but seizures appear in the first year of life.

Answer 292
A True Using glucose metabolism in brain to detect and localise metabolic changes associated with seizures.
B True Can be used in three phases: ictal, interictal and postictal.
C True Localisation of brain language and motor area.
D False No longer in use as it causes side effects.
E False

Answer 293
A False Can be worsened with carbamazepine. Best treatment is sodium valproate, lamotrigine or topiramate.
B True Should not be used in children except in those with infantile spasm, especially secondary to TS.
C True Also sodium valproate.
D True Can also be used in generalised seizures.
E True Also effective in 60% of partial seizures.

Answer 294
A True From disturbance of cardiac rhythm, mainly in young adults.
B False It is about 30%.
C True Patients without neurological impairment who suffer from any form of epilepsy do less well than normal population.
D False Patients who remain seizure free for 2–3 years will have a lower risk of relapse.
E False They are enzyme inducers and should be increased by at least 30%.

Answer 295
A True As well as pizotifen.
B True Considered to be the drug of choice by some neurologists but has many side effects.
C True May cause low blood pressure.
D True Also methysergide.
E True As a vasodilator.

Answer 296
A True
B True
C False
D False
E False

Answer 297

A True
B True
C True
D False
E False

Answer 298

A False
B True
C False
D True   Also penicillinamine and carnitine.
E False   It is used to treat myasthenia.

Infectious diseases answers

Answer 299
A True
B False Chicken pox and measles are caused by herpes viruses.
C False Rubella is caused by a togavirus and poliomyelitis is caused by an enterovirus.
D False HIV is a retrovirus; type I causes AIDS. Hepatitis A is caused by a picornavirus.
E True

Answer 300
A True
B False It is usually vesicular.
C False Maculopapular.
D False Echoviruses may cause a telangiectatic rash.
E False Maculopapular.

Answer 301
A False Gram-negative.
B True
C True Shigella, *Haemophilus influenzae*, Pneumococcus, staphylococci and *Mycobacterium tuberculosis* are Gram-positive.
D False Gram-negative.
E False Gram-negative.

Answer 302
A True
B False It has 40 different antigenic proteins.
C False
D False The toxin is responsible for the rash.
E True

Answer 303
A False Usually after the neonatal period.
B True
C True
D True
E False May cause meningitis but it is not common.

Answer 304

A False
B True
C True
D True   *Haemophilus influenzae* type b, *Streptococcus pneumoniae* and *Neisseria meningitidis* are the commonest causes of meningitis in children between the ages of 2 months and 12 years.
E False   This may cause meningitis in children with immunological problems, as may *Pseudomonas aeruginosa*, *Staphylococcus aureus*, Salmonella and *Listeria monocytogenes*.

Answer 305

A False   It is a Gram-positive bacillus.
B True   This inhibits protein synthesis and causes local tissue necrosis.
C False   The strongest is gravis.
D False   Antitoxin will not neutralise the free toxin.
E True   It can cause skin and mucosal infection.

Answer 306

A True
B False   It can produce exotoxin.
C True
D False   In generalised tetanus, trismus (lockjaw) is the presenting symptom in >50% of patients. This is followed by stiffness, muscle spasm and dysphagia.
E False   This is given intramuscularly.

Answer 307

A True
B False
C False
D True
E True

Answer 308

A False   It is Gram-negative.
B False   It can affect all ages but classically occurs in the younger age group (<1 year of age).
C False   They are usually 2 weeks apart.
D False   It usually occurs in the paroxysmal stage.
E True   Only if it is given early.

Answer 309
A True
B True
C True
D True
E True

Answer 310
A True   It is done by giving the PPD intradermally.
B False   It is a type IV hypersensitivity reaction.
C False   There is a delayed reaction of more than 72 hours at a young age, in miliary TB, malnutrition, infection with measles, rubella, mumps, influenza and live virus vaccines. It is negative if there is poor technique or the results are misread.
D False   1:10000 and also 1:100.
E True

Answer 311
A False   This is associated with tuberculoid leprosy; the lesion is also hypopigmented, atrophic and flat. The closest superficial nerve is often thick.
B True
C True
D True
E True   There is loss of the eyebrows, anaesthesia of the lesions is mild and symmetrical peripheral sensory neuropathy is common. Azoospermia, infertility and gynaecomastia are common in adults only.

Answer 312
A False   The bacillus is Gram-negative; fresh water is the environmental reservoir.
B True   Hyponatraemia, hypophosphataemia, abnormal liver function and renal dysfunction are other extrapulmonary manifestations.
C False
D False
E True

Answer 313
A True
B False   Otitis media, pneumonia and encephalomyelitis are common.
C True
D False   This may occur between 6 months and 6 years after measles infection.
E True   An infrequent serious complication.

Answer 314

A True   They usually occur following the prodromal phase. They are usually seen opposite the lower molars.

B False   More than 80% will show antibodies.

C False   Cervical and suboccipital lymph gland enlargement.

D False   It is not common; it may follow rubella infection.

E False   Chicken pox or varicella is associated with lifelong immunity.

Answer 315

A False   A child may develop chicken pox when exposed to shingles.

B True

C False   Pain, hyperaesthesia, pruritus and low grade fever may precede or accompany the dermatomal vesicular lesion.

D True

E False   Unusual in children.

Answer 316

A False

B False   It can be caused by parainfluenza, adeno- and influenza viruses.

C True

D False   This usually follows Coxsackie A virus infection.

E False   This may be caused by adenovirus.

Answer 317

A True   The rash is macular rose spots or maculopapular. It appears on about the seventh to tenth day.

B True

C False   First appears on trunk.

D False   It lasts for only 2–3 days.

E True

Answer 318

A True

B False   It is associated with arthralgia and diarrhoea.

C False

D True   Especially with hepatitis C.

E True

Answer 319

A True

B False   There is no need to repeat the test and the person should be vaccinated again.

C False   The rate of success is 90%.

D False

E False   There is a vaccine.

Answer 320

A True

B True

C True From lying in bed.

D False

E True

Answer 321

A False It can be used for influenza.

B True

C False

D True

E False It can be used for CMV infection.

Answer 322

A False Caused by Gram-negative bacilli (*Rochalimaea quintana* and *henselae*).

B True It follows direct contact with cats, dogs and monkeys.

C False Extensive lymphadenopathy is the commonest feature; the patient may have fever, malaise, headache, and anorexia.

D True

E False No antimicrobial therapy is required. Surgical removal is the best option; fine needle aspiration or surgical biopsy will cause fistula and tissue granulation.

Answer 323

A False Isolated from stool.

B True

C True

D True

E False It is not associated with diarrhoea.

Answer 324

A True

B False For strongyloidosis, thiabendazole and ivermectin can be used in children. For ascariasis, piperazine salts can be used.

C False Hook worms can be treated with mebendazole.

D True

E True It is also used in schistosomiasis.

Dermatology answers

Answer 325

A True Harlequin colour changes, naevus simplex, mongolian blue spot, transient pustular melanosis and sebaceous hyperplasia are other neonatal rashes that usually disappear; no treatment is required.

B True This occurs when a newborn baby is exposed to low environmental temperature.

C False

D True

E False

Answer 326

A False Emulsified creams and special shampoo and, sometimes, hydrocortisone can be used.

B True

C False Zinc with castor oil is effective and helps to keep it dry.

D False Nystatin or miconazole is effective in candidiasis.

E True

Answer 327

A False It is usually epidermal oedema.

B True

C False In 90% of affected children, eczema has usually disappeared by the age of 16 years.

D True

E False

Answer 328

A True

B False Peutz–Jeghers syndrome is characterised by mucosal pigmentation of the lips and gums, and hamartomas of the stomach and small bowel. It is inherited as autosomal dominant.

C False This is associated with Crohn's disease.

D True

E True

Answer 329

A False   It is used in treatment of acne.
B True   Phenytoin, phenobarbital, lithium, androgens and vitamin B_{12} can cause acne.
C False
D True
E False

Answer 330

A True   Fungal infection, trauma, psoriasis, cosmetics, vincristine, bleomycin, indomethacin, tetracycline and porphyria are causes of separation of the nail plate from the distal nail bed.
B False
C True   Vasculitis, trauma, severe rheumatoid arthritis, peptic ulcer disease, cirrhosis, glomerulonephritis, scurvy, trichinosis, malignant disease and psoriasis are causes of splinter haemorrhage.
D True
E True

Answer 331

A True
B False   Seborrhoeic dermatitis can affect any age and its cause is unknown.
C True
D True
E False   Antiseborrhoeic shampoo is useful for scalp lesions.

Answer 332

A True   Chronic constipation and soiling, poor hygiene, repeated UTI and allergy to materials are causes of vulvovaginitis in girls.
B True
C False
D True
E True

Answer 333

A False   Poxvirus.
B False   Human papillomaviruses.
C True
D False   *Staphylococcus aureus* and streptococci.
E False   Herpes virus.

Answer 334

A True There are many causes of urticaria, which is mostly mediated by IgE.
B True
C True
D True
E True

Answer 335

A False Pityriasis versicolor is caused by *Pityrosporum orbiculare*.
B False Streptococcal infection.
C True
D False *Staphylococcus aureus* infection.
E False Tinea versicolor is caused by *Malassezia furfur*, and tinea capitis by *Trichophyton*.

Answer 336

A False
B False Extensor areas.
C True
D True Face and proximal portions of limbs.
E True

Answer 337

A False It is associated with cavernous haemangioma.
B True
C True
D False
E True It is associated with cavernous haemangioma.

Answer 338

A True Risk factors for melanoma are presence of familial atypical mole–melanoma syndrome, xeroderma pigmentosum, increased number of melanocytic naevi, excessive sun exposure, family history of melanoma and immunosuppression.
B True
C False
D True
E False

Answer 339
A False   Hard nodules.
B False   Firm nodules.
C True
D True
E False   Cystic nodules.

Answer 340
A True
B False   Albinism, tuberous sclerosis, hypomelanosis of Ito, Waardenburg's syndrome, Chediak–Higashi syndrome and vitiligo are associated with hypopigmentation.
C True
D True
E True

Answer 341
A True
B False   It is associated with hair being pulled out.
C True
D False   It is X-linked recessive.
E True

Answer 342
A True
B False   Autosomal dominant.
C False   Autosomal recessive.
D True
E True

Answer 343
A True
B True
C False
D True
E False   It is associated with precocious puberty, polyostotic fibrous dysplasia and abnormal pigmentation.

Answer 344
A False   They are involved in allergy.
B True
C False   They are constituents of epidermis.
D False   Epidermis.
E True

Joint and bone diseases answers

Answer 345

A False   In systemic onset, RF and ANA are negative; there is leukocytosis, severe anaemia, hepatosplenomegaly, pleuritis or pericarditis, iridocyclitis, arthritis and rheumatoid rash.

B False   Rheumatoid factor is only positive in polyarticular JCA in girls.

C True   This is associated with pauci-articular type I. Polyarticular JCA with positive rheumatoid factor also shows presence of ANA in 75% of cases.

D True

E True   It is associated with pauci-articular type II.

Answer 346

A False   Bowing of the legs can be found in normal infants, especially when they start to walk

B True   There is lack of calcification of osteoid (osteopenia). In the wrist, X-ray appearances include widening of the growth plate and splaying and cupping of the epiphysis.

C True

D False

E False

Answer 347

A True

B False   Septic arthritis, Lyme disease, osteomyelitis, JCA, SLE, Kawasaki vasculitis and dermatomyositis can cause acute arthritis.

C False

D True

E True

Answer 348

A False   It can affect boys.

B False   It is only bilateral in a few cases (20%).

C True   This is the classical presentation. There is mild restriction of abduction and internal rotation of thigh and mild shortness of stature. Cessation of femoral epiphysis growth, subchondral fracture, fragmentation, reossification and healed stage are the X-ray appearances.

D False

E True

Answer 349

A False   Takayasu arteritis is rare. It is an inflammatory process involving the aorta and its branches. It may affect kidneys, brain and eyes.

B True

C True

D False   Takayasu arteritis.

E True

Answer 350

A True   The ESR, CRP, white cell count and neutrophils are high. The synovial fluid is purulent with a high white cell count, and Gram stain is positive in 50%.

B True

C False   The glucose content is low.

D False   This is done if joint aspiration is negative and to diagnose osteomyelitis.

E True

Answer 351

A True   Non-osseous causes are Sandifer's syndrome, gastro-oesophageal reflux and posterior fossa and spinal cord tumours. Osseous causes are atlas malformation, congenital cervical scoliosis, rotatory fixation of C1–C2, trauma, upper respiratory infection and cervical adenitis. Sternomastoid injury causes torticollis in newborn babies.

B True

C False

D True

E True

Answer 352

A True   Hepatosplenomegaly and lymphadenopathy occur in most children, only one-third have pericarditis or pleuritis, and a few children have abdominal pain. Systemic onset JCA is characterised by high temperature twice a day and a rheumatoid rash.

B False

C True

D False   The ESR and CRP are usually elevated, but not always; they can be normal. ANA and RF are negative in systemic onset JCA. All serum immunoglobulin levels are elevated.

E False

Answer 353

A True   Similar to salicylate side effects. All NSAIDs may exacerbate asthma.

B False

C True   Gastritis, raised level of liver enzymes, bleeding and Reye's syndrome should be considered as side effects of salicylates.

D True

E True

Answer 354

A True

B True

C False   It is associated with polyarteritis nodosa.

D True

E False   It is associated with polyarteritis nodosa, scleroderma and systemic sclerosis.

Answer 355

A True   Bilateral non-purulent conjunctival injection, infected or dry fissured lips, oedema or erythema of hands and feet, truncal polymorphic and non-vesicular rash, and cervical lymphadenopathy. Four of these plus fever lasting for at least 5 days are diagnostic criteria of Kawasaki disease.

B True

C True

D False

E False

Answer 356

A True

B True

C True

D True   Also Marfan's syndrome.

E True

Answer 357

A True   It is usually inherited as autosomal dominant.

B False   Decrease in lumbar interpedicular distance.

C True

D False   Hydrocephalus is common.

E True

Answer 358

A True   It is also associated with ASD and dwarfism.
B True   Also renal defect.
C True   Also blindness with dwarfism.
D True   Also atrophic terminal phalanges.
E True   Also fever with irritability.

Answer 359

A False   Polydactyly.
B True
C False
D True
E False   Broad thumb.

Eyes, ears, nose and throat answers

Answer 360

A False
B True
C False May be associated with cataract.
D True
E True Scheie, Morquio, Maroteaux–Lamy and Sly syndromes, generalised gangliosidosis and Fabry's disease are associated with corneal deposition.

Answer 361

A True Galactokinase deficiency, hypocalcaemia, IDDM, Lowe's syndrome and Niemann–Pick disease can be associated with cataract.
B True
C True Trisomies 13, 18, and Turner's syndrome.
D True
E False

Answer 362

A False It is usually unilateral.
B False Visual acuity is usually normal.
C True Amblyopia is usually asymptomatic and detected by screening programme.
D True If not treated early.
E True If it is severe.

Answer 363

A True It may also be associated with diphtheria, diabetes mellitus, syphilis and oculomotor nerve lesions.
B True
C True
D False Ptosis is associated with astigmatism.
E True

Answer 364

A True
B False
C True It is also associated with micro-opthalmia, corneal opacification, dense cataract, chorioretinal scars, macular defect, retinal dysplasia and severe optic nerve hypoplasia. In older children who once had useful vision it may be due to cataract, chorioretinitis, retinoblastoma and retinitis pigmentosa.
D True
E True

Answer 365

A True
B False
C True
D False
E True

Answer 366

A False It is on adduction.
B True
C False It is acquired abducens nerve palsy.
D False It is vertical gaze palsy.
E False Elevation of the eye in adduction position is reduced or absent.

Answer 367

A True
B False It is usually after the first 48 hours.
C False Immediately after application, not congenital.
D True
E True

Answer 368

A False Children with lens subluxation may present with blurring vision as myopia or astigmatism.
B False It is upward and outward.
C True Uveitis, intraocular tumour, congenital glaucoma, high myopia, and cataract are associated with lens displacement.
D True
E False It may follow megalocornea.

Answer 369

A False   The vision defect varies with the nature and site of the primary disease or lesion.

B True

C True   Intracranial tumours, hereditary disorders (AD, AR), trauma, degenerative and inflammatory diseases are associated with optic atrophy.

D True

E False

Answer 370

A True

B True

C False   Group A beta-haemolytic streptococcus.

D True

E False

Answer 371

A True   Craniofacial anomalies, ototoxic medication (aminoglycosides) and dysmorphic features associated with hearing loss are also indications for neonatal screening for hearing loss.

B True

C True

D True

E True

Answer 372

A True

B True

C True

D False   Response to Stycar picture is usually at 3 years.

E True

Answer 373

A True   Pain is the commonest feature; conductive hearing loss may occur.

B True

C False   This is a feature of acute otitis media.

D False

E True

Answer 374

A False Maxillary.
B True
C False Headache is usually uncommon.
D True
E False Sinus CT is most likely to be used in diagnosing chronic
         sinusitis.

Oncology answers

Answer 375

  A True

  B True

  C True

  D True   May be due to biliary obstruction.

  E True   May be due to mediastinal lymphadenopathy or chest infection with effusion.

Answer 376

  A True   The karyotypes of leukaemic cells have diagnostic, prognostic and therapeutic significance.

  B True

  C False   There is little cytoplasm in L1, L2 has more cytoplasm, and L3 has prominent nucleoli and deep blue cytoplasm with prominent vacuolisation.

  D False

  E True

Answer 377

  A False   AML constitutes 15–20% of all childhood leukaemia in children under the age of 15 years. It should be considered in children presenting with temperature, malaise, frequent bruising, pallor and large liver and spleen.

  B True

  C False   It is not a common presentation; neither is bone pain.

  D True

  E False   At least 30% of leukaemic blast cells should be present in bone marrow to diagnose AML.

Answer 378

  A False   FAB lists 8 subtypes from M0 to M7. M0 to M7 account for 80% of childhood AML.

  B False

  C False

  D True

  E True

Answer 379

A True
B True   Nodular sclerosing is the commonest form, accounting for 50% of cases in children and 70% in adolescents. The mixed cellularity form is second and accounts for 40–50% of patients. The lymphocyte predominant variety affects 20–30% and has a very good prognosis. The lymphocyte depleted variety affects 10% of patients and has a poor prognosis.
C True   Lymph nodes are painless, enlarged, firm, non-tender and usually discrete.
D True
E True

Answer 380

A True   Secondary bone metastasis.
B False
C True
D False
E False

Answer 381

A False   Involvement of two or more lymphoid regions on the same side of the diaphragm.
B True
C True   Radiotherapy is very effective for localised stage I and IIA disease in patients who have achieved their full growth. Other stages may benefit from the combination of radio- and chemotherapy.
D True
E True

Answer 382

A False   It is a malignant clonal proliferation of primarily T or B lymphocytes.
B False   Abdominal mass is the most frequent presentation; 30% of patients present with cervical lymphadenopathy, and 30% with mediastinal mass.
C True   Also thrombocytopenia, which is due to bone marrow involvement.
D True
E True   Approximately 70% for those with stage III and IV.

Answer 383
A False The insulin level is high even when there is hypoglycaemia.
B True Absence of ketonaemia, acidosis, and elevated C-peptide at the time of hypoglycaemia are other features of hyperinsulinaemia.
C True
D True
E False Subtotal pancreatectomy is the treatment of choice for insulinoma.

Answer 384
A True
B False
C True
D False
E True

Answer 385
A False Intrathecal administration and radiotherapy are good ways to treat CNS involvement.
B False There may be short stature, secondary malignancy and infertility.
C True
D False Facial palsy may be due to leukaemia or radiotherapy.
E False The commonest site of relapse is the bone marrow.

Answer 386
A True There is bone involvement in 80%; bilateral exophthalmos is also present with pituitary dysfunction and diabetes insipidus. Systemic manifestations of fever, weight loss and anaemia or thrombocytopenia are other presenting features.
B True Or petechial in appearance.
C False
D True
E False Several different regimens are used in disseminated disease.

Answer 387
A True Is very effective for localised tumour.
B False Several different regimens are used in disseminated disease.
C False All neuroblastomas are radiosensitive.
D True It is also used as a diagnostic procedure.
E False

Answer 388

A True   WAGR syndrome (Wilms', aniridia, genitourinary malformation and mental retardation).

B True   Denys–Dras syndrome (Wilms', nephropathy, and genital abnormalities). It is also associated with Beckwith–Wiedemann syndrome. It can be familial in 30% of patients.

C False Deletions involve one of at least two loci on chromosome 11.

D True

E False

Answer 389

A True   The most common presenting feature.

B True

C True

D True   Due to extensive bone involvement.

E True   Sarcoma botryoides.

Answer 390

A True

B True   Chemotherapy can be used after surgery or if secondary metastasis occurs.

C True

D True

E False Has no role in retinoblastoma. The finding of leukocoria, which is a yellowish white reflex in the pupil, on detailed eye examination is an indication.

Community paediatrics answers

Answer 391

A True

B True   Most incidental skull fractures affect the temporal bone.

C True   Shaken baby syndrome, which is also associated with subdural bleeding in most cases.

D False

E True   This is the commonest location of cigarette burning.

Answer 392

A False   If UTI is frequent this may raise the suspicion of CSA.

B False

C False   This is usually accidental when trying to zip or unzip trousers.

D True   Also vaginal bleeding in preschool girls or evidence of sexually transmitted diseases.

E False

Answer 393

A False   The abuser is usually a member of the family. Father or sibling is more frequently the abuser than the stepfather.

B False   It is becoming more common and boys are usually abused more than girls.

C True   Full examination of any physically abused child is required.

D True   As in many papers published by Dr C Hobbs.

E False   Disclosure is very important in CSA.

Answer 394

A True

B True

C True

D False

E False

Answer 395

A False   Can be held for other reasons, e.g. neonatal unit, handicapped child.

B True

C False   He or she should attend.

D False   Parents should always be invited.

E False

Answer 396

A False   7–10 days.
B False   Describe what you see and write down only the facts.
C False   There is no need to take the notes. You may lose them and evidence may change.
D False   A carer may be present or the child may choose a nurse or social worker. Always ask someone to chaperone you when examining a child suspected of having been sexually abused.
E True

Answer 397

A False
B True
C True
D True
E False   A student test is more sensitive.

Answer 398

A True   Variance is the sum of the squares of the differences from the mean, divided by the number of observations minus one.
B False   1 SD ± mean = 68%. 2 SD means that 95% of values fall within that range, and 3 SD gives 99.73% confidence limits.
C False   Chi-square compares frequency of a variable in two populations.
D True
E False   SD is useful in the interpretation of data in terms of probability only if the population forms a normal distribution.

Answer 399

A True
B False
C False   Abdominal ultrasound can be done to look for any renal problem or bladder abnormality and also to measure the residual volume.
D False   They may be bullied at school but generally they do very well.
E False   Reduction of fluid intake at night, star chart, bell, and psychologist and nurse specialist should be tried. If all these fail, then drugs such as imipramine, desmopressin and oxybutynin can be used.

Answer 400

A True
B True
C True
D False
E True A marker study can be done to assess gut motility and to show the child that there is no problem with their gut. Various regimens of laxative can be tried, and admission for one day may be indicated in severe cases to clean them up.

Answer 401

A True Drugs taken by the breast-feeding mother during pregnancy should not be stopped at all as the baby is used to swimming in fluid full of these drugs. If lactating women take any drug, only about 10% will be secreted in the milk. Some drugs should be avoided or alternative ones can be given to breast-feeding mothers.
B True This should be avoided.
C False
D True
E True

Answer 402

A True
B True
C False May be avoided as it may cause drowsiness in the baby if the mother is on high doses.
D True
E False

Answer 403

A False May cause failure to thrive but not feeding problems.
B False
C False
D True Other causes of feeding problems in newborn babies include first baby, retracted nipples, poor milk production, using an unsuitable teat for the bottle-fed babies, cleft lip and palate and choanal atresia. Such babies often present with failure to regain birthweight at 2 or 3 weeks of age.
E True

Mock exam questions

Question 1

The incidence of psychiatric disease is increased in the following

    A Socially deprived inner city area
    B Adopted child
    C Child of divorced parents
    D Moderately severe learning difficulty
    E Severely physically disabled child

Question 2

Characteristic features of Marfan's syndrome

    A Associated with spontaneous mutation in 50% of cases
    B Associated with hypercalcaemia in 20% of cases
    C Lens subluxation is downward
    D Pulmonary stenosis is common
    E High arched palate

Question 3

In a normal adolescent, BP is reduced

    A During sleep
    B On standing
    C On inspiration
    D On exercise
    E On smoking

Question 4

Metabolic acidosis occurs in

    A Ethanol poisoning
    B Chronic renal failure
    C Sodium valproate poisoning
    D Salicylate poisoning
    E Pancreatic fistula

Question 5

Defective cellular immunity causes a negative tuberculin test in patients with

A Tuberculosis
B Hodgkin's lymphoma
C Thymic aplasia
D Sarcoidosis
E Vaccination with live virus

Question 6

In Down's syndrome, the incidence of the following conditions can be increased

A Coeliac disease
B Alzheimer's disease
C Acute leukaemia
D Cervical spondylosis
E Cervical vertebral dislocation

Question 7

Common features of infectious mononucleosis include

A Petechial haemorrhage of the palate
B Abdominal pain
C Peeling of skin
D Inflamed tonsils
E Strawberry tongue appearance

Question 8

Infection with *Giardia lamblia*

A Absence of cysts excludes the diagnosis
B Causes acute blood loss
C Causes total villous atrophy
D Causes malabsorption
E Is associated with cow's milk intolerance

Question 9

Von Willibrand's disease is characterised by

A Increased BT
B Decreased TT
C Defective platelet aggregation
D Platelet aggregation with ristocetin
E Autosomal dominant

Question 10

A normal 6-month-old infant

- A Demonstrates a Moro reflex
- B Rolls from back onto front
- C Holds an object between index finger and thumb
- D Has good head control
- E Responds to a distraction test

Question 11

Ingestion of ecstasy may lead to

- A Convulsion
- B Hepatic failure
- C Hyperthermia
- D Increase in CK
- E Cerebral haemorrhage

Question 12

Tonsillar exudate may be associated with

- A Kawasaki disease
- B Epstein–Barr virus infection
- C AIDS
- D Measles
- E Herpes virus infection

Question 13

A diagnosis of pulmonary stenosis rather than ASD can be made if there is

- A RBBB on ECG
- B Parasternal heave
- C Fixed splitting of the second heart sound
- D Early ejection systolic click
- E Right ventricular hypertrophy

Question 14

Are the following statements about juvenile chronic arthritis true or false?

A Associated with microcytic hypochromic anaemia due to iron depletion
B ANA are commonly positive
C Normal radiography excludes the diagnosis
D Ophthalmological review is not necessary
E Can be familial

Question 15

In a 3-week-old baby presenting with persistent vomiting, the conditions to be considered are

A Duodenal atresia
B Pyloric stenosis
C Gastero-esophageal reflux
D Sepsis
E Overfeeding

Question 16

Live vaccines include

A Hib
B Measles
C Tetanus
D Polio
E BCG

Question 17

Lower GIT bleeding is a common association with

A Shigella dysentery
B Crohn's disease
C Giardiasis
D Intussusception
E Constipation

Question 18

In cystic fibrosis

A Infertility is more common in males
B Hepatic fibrosis is an early finding
C The incidence is 1 in 20 000 of population in the northern hemisphere
D One-third of patients present with meconium ileus
E The delta 508 deletion is the most common

Question 19

Varicella zoster immunoglobulin is indicated for

A A mother who contracted chicken pox in early pregnancy
B A steroid-dependent asthmatic with a history of chicken pox contact
C Immunosuppressed patients without a history of contact
D Those travelling to highly endemic areas
E Patients with severe atopic eczema

Question 20

Duchenne muscular dystrophy

A May present as floppiness at birth
B Children who are delayed in walking by 18 months of age need to have CK measured
C EMG has no place in diagnosing DMD
D May be associated with IDDM
E All cases are inherited as X-linked dominant

Question 21

The following suggest prerenal rather than renal failure

A Urine to plasma urea ratio increased to 1.5
B Urinary sodium >40 mmol/l
C Urine to plasma osmolality ratio increased by 2.5
D Fractional excretion of sodium >1
E Urinary output is >1 ml/kg/h

Question 22

The following are non-physiological findings

A In term babies, hyperbilirubinaemia >150 at 20 hours of age
B BP of 120/80 in a 5-year-old
C Random glucose of 15 mmol/l in a 10-year-old girl
D Hb of 11.5 g/dl in a 1-year-old boy
E BMI of 20 in an 11-year-old

Question 23

These are the commonest causes of neonatal seizures

A Maternal hypothyroidism
B Pyridoxine deficiency
C Polycythaemia
D Sepsis
E Hypoglycaemia

Question 24

Appendicitis in a preschool child

A The diagnosis can be excluded if there is no peritonitis
B Abdominal US is helpful in diagnosis
C Normal WCC can exclude the diagnosis
D Becomes perforated more often in a child than in an adolescent
E Mainly associated with Henoch–Schönlein purpura

Question 25

These conditions may cause long-term effects

A PKU
B Treated aortic coarctation
C Hepatitis A 10 years before
D Treated ALL with remission after 5 years
e Treated UTI

Question 26

The following nerves contain preganglionic parasympathetic fibres as they leave the brain

A Oculomotor
B Trigeminal
C Facial
D Vagus
E Hypoglossus

Question 27

The following disorders can be identified by gene location in most patients

A Cystic fibrosis
B Huntington's chorea
C Muscular dystrophy
D Pyloric stenosis
E Lennox–Gastaut syndrome

Question 28

Parathyroid hormones may be low in

A CHARG syndrome
B DiGeorge syndrome
C Nutritional rickets
D Hypophosphataemic rickets
E Hypothyroidism

Question 29

The following require referral to a child psychiatrist

A A child with a headache for the last 3 months
B A toddler who is failing to thrive
C A daydreamer
D A 3-year-old child who does not mix with others
E A 3-year-old child who does not want to stay with her family

Question 30

Characteristic features of childhood autism are

A Abnormal EEG
B Lack of eye to eye contact
C Ritual behaviour
D Delayed language development
E Abnormal hand movement

Question 31

In WPW syndrome, the following are true

A Digoxin is the drug of choice for cardiac arrhythmia
B Prolonged PR interval
C Associated with ASD
D Only present during infancy
E No benefit from surgical correction

Question 32

Nocturnal seizures are a manifestation of

A Landu–Kleffner syndrome
B Benign Rolandic epilepsy of childhood
C Hypopituitarism
D Glycogen storage disease type Ia
E Temporal lobe epilepsy syndrome

Question 33

Hyposplenism is associated with

A Portal hypertension
B Sickle cell disease
C Addison's disease
D Pneumococcal sepsis
E Coeliac disease

Question 34

Are the following statements about IgE true or false?

A It crosses the placenta
B It is responsible for type II hypersensitivity reactions
C It is involved in anaphylactic reactions
D It is present in blood in the same amount as plasma IgG
E Levels may be high during sepsis

Question 35

Corneal opacities are a recognised feature of

A Hurler's syndrome
B Congenital CMV infection
C Marfan's syndrome
D Osteogenesis imperfecta
E Hyperparathyroidism

Question 36

Are the following statements about herpes encephalitis true or false?

A It can be caused by type II herpes virus
B The EEG is abnormal even when cranial CT is normal
C It may lead to epilepsy
D CSF will show lymphocytosis and low glucose
E 2 weeks of IV acyclovir and 2 weeks of oral acyclovir is the treatment of choice

Question 37

Cleft lip and palate can be associated with

A Deafness
B Micrognathia
C Maternal anticonvulsant therapy
D Inability to breast-feed
E Upper airway obstruction

Question 38

Fragile X syndrome is characterised by

A Large head
B Large penis
C Coarctation of aorta
D Only males affected
E Mental retardation in 10% of cases

Question 39

Jejunal villi are characterised by

A Intraepithelial lymphocytes
B Neuroepithelial cells
C Total atrophy with cow's milk intolerance
D No secretory cells among the other cells
E Being the commonest site for tape worms

Question 40

Are the following associations true or false?

A Carbamazepine—juvenile myoclonic epilepsy
B Phenytoin—G6PD
C Williams' syndrome—pulmonary stenosis
D Leptospirosis—gentamicin
E Nitrous oxide—pulmonary hypertension

Question 41

Which of the following are good clinical markers of CSA?

A Anogenital warts
B Anal fissure
C UTI in girls
D Herpes simplex vaginitis
E Laceration of penis

Question 42

Minimal change glomerulonephritis is characterised by

A Hypertension
B Haematuria
C Proteinuria
D Reduced C3 level
E Increased ANA level

Question 43

Microscopic haematuria occurs in the following conditions

A IgA nephropathy
B Cyclosporine nephrotoxicity
C Membranous glomerulonephropathy
D HSP
E Trauma

Question 44

Recognised features of Turner's syndrome are

A Horseshoe kidney
B Peripheral pulmonary stenosis
C Lymphoedema
D Hypertension
E Psychosis

Question 45

The following are produced by ectoderm

A Skin
B Liver
C Hair
D Radial nerve
E Tongue

Question 46

Indications for renal biopsy in a 10-year-old child with nephrotic syndrome are

A Microscopic haematuria
B Serum albumin of <10 g/dl
C Persistent low level of C3
D Creatinine >200 mmol/l
E SLE

Question 47

Coeliac disease

A Anaemia is due to folic acid deficiency
B Is associated with ankylosing spondylitis
C Presents in early childhood
D Is associated with GIT lymphoma
E Is associated with mouth ulcers

Question 48

Congenital hip dislocation

A Male > female
B Is associated with breech presentation
C May be responsible for delay in walking
D Diagnosis made by hip X-ray at 1 week of age
E Could be due to intrauterine infection

Question 49

Are the following statements about atopic eczema true or false?

A It presents at birth
B Extensor surfaces are more affected than flexural
C Treated by UV light
D Gets better with age
E More common in breast-fed babies

Question 50

Are the following statements true or false?

A The muscles of the thenar eminence are supplied solely by the median nerve
B Paralysis of lateral popliteal nerve causes loss of ankle jerks
C Injury to the radial nerve causes loss of the first dorsal interosseus
D Sciatic nerve damage causes loss of dorsiflexion
E Femoral nerve damage causes adductor paralysis

Question 51

Prader–Willi syndrome

A In 50% of cases is associated with deletion of maternal chromosome 15
B Is associated with scoliosis
C Excessive weight is easily managed with diet
D Is associated with big hands
E Is associated with persistent hypotonia

Question 52

The following drugs can be given to a child with mild renal failure

A Paracetamol
B Nitrofurantoin
C Salbutamol
D Captopril
E Fluconazole

Question 53

Scrotal tenderness in 6-year-old child may be due to

A Indirect inguinal hernia
B Torsion of the testis
C Phlebitis
D Nephrotic syndrome
E Sickle cell crisis

Question 54

The following conditions are inherited as autosomal dominant

A Vitamin D resistant rickets
B Ataxia telangiectasia
C Hereditary spherocytosis
D Pyloric stenosis
E Incontinentia pigmenti

Question 55

Membranous nephropathy

A C3 is low
B There is no association with haematuria
C Is the commonest nephropathy associated with SLE
D May be caused by helmintic infection
E Is associated with normal blood pressure

Question 56

Poor prognostic features of ALL are

A Age <2 or >10 years
B Male
C High white cell count on presentation
D cALL type
E Abnormal clotting

Question 57

Poor prognostic features in meningococcaemia are

A High WCC
B Purpuric rashes on the face
C High temperature
D Renal failure
E Convulsions

Question 58

Hormonal changes associated with anorexia nervosa are

A High GH
B Low FSH
C High cortisol
D Low oestradiol
E Normal TSH

Question 59

DNA repair can be associated with the following conditions

A Epidermolysis bullosa
B Ataxia telangiectasia
C Fanconi's anaemia
D Xeroderma pigmentosum
E Sturge–Weber syndrome

Question 60

Steroids can be used as a treatment in

A Croup
B Herpes simplex corneal ulcers
C Acute disseminated encephalomyelitis
D Cystic fibrosis
E ITP

Answers to mock exam questions

1	T	F	T	F	T	21	F	T	F	T	T	41	T	F	F	T	F
2	T	F	F	F	T	22	T	F	T	F	F	42	F	T	T	T	F
3	T	T	F	F	F	23	F	T	F	T	T	43	T	T	T	T	T
4	T	T	F	T	F	24	F	T	F	T	F	44	T	F	T	T	T
5	F	T	T	T	T	25	T	T	F	T	F	45	T	F	T	T	F
6	F	T	T	F	T	26	T	F	T	F	F	46	F	F	T	T	T
7	T	T	F	T	F	27	T	T	T	F	F	47	F	F	F	T	T
8	F	T	F	F	F	28	F	T	F	F	F	48	F	T	T	F	T
9	T	F	F	T	T	29	F	F	F	T	F	49	F	T	F	T	F
10	F	T	F	T	F	30	F	T	T	T	F	50	F	T	F	T	F
11	T	T	T	T	T	31	F	F	F	F	F	51	F	F	F	F	F
12	F	T	F	F	F	32	T	T	T	T	F	52	T	T	T	T	T
13	F	T	F	T	F	33	F	T	F	F	F	53	T	T	T	F	T
14	F	F	F	F	T	34	F	F	F	F	T	54	F	F	T	F	F
15	F	T	T	T	T	35	F	F	F	F	F	55	F	F	F	T	T
16	F	T	F	T	T	36	T	T	T	F	T	56	T	T	T	F	F
17	T	T	T	T	T	37	T	T	T	T	F	57	T	F	F	T	T
18	T	F	T	T	T	38	F	T	F	F	F	58	T	T	T	T	T
19	F	F	F	F	F	39	T	T	F	F	F	59	F	T	T	T	F
20	T	T	F	T	F	40	F	F	F	F	T	60	T	F	T	F	T